The Executive's Guide to Health and Fitness

by *Kenneth H. Franklin*

Illustrated by Robert Bugg

Published by The Economics Press, Inc.
12 Daniel Road, Fairfield, N.J. 07006

This book is about getting and staying healthy. We believe the advice it contains is correct, sound, and reasonable. But because each of us has differing capabilities, needs, and goals, we recommend you consult with your physician before commencing any program of exercise.

Copyright © 1985, The Economics Press, Inc., Fairfield, N.J. 07006

All inquiries should be addressed to The Economics Press, Inc., 12 Daniel Road, Fairfield, N.J. 07006

ISBN 0-910187-04-5
Printed in the United States of America

Table of Contents

Acknowledgments...7

Foreword..9

Section I - Exercise...12

Chapter 1: Why You Hate Exercise
  (And What to Do About It)....................................14

Chapter 2: The Best Thing Since Sliced Bread...............17

Chapter 3: How Much Exercise Is Enough?...................20

Chapter 4: Exercise Palaces: Welcome to the Club!.........22

Chapter 5: Running—the Fad That Never Faded...........25

Chapter 6: The More It's Fun, the More You'll Run.......28

Chapter 7: Walking—It's Better Than You Think..........31

Chapter 8: Cycling: One Wheel or Two?......................34

Which Exercises Are Best?.......................................37

Before the Run—Stretching Those Muscles...................40

Section II - Nutrition & Weight Control......................44

Chapter 9: Food—the Good Guys and the Bad Guys.......46

Chapter 10: Pizza for Breakfast?...............................50

Chapter 11: Snacks That Are Good for You..................53

Chapter 12: What's So Good About Fiber?...................56

Chapter 13: Salad Bars: What to Pick.........................59

Chapter 14: Is Fast Food the Same As Junk Food?.........62

Chapter 15: Caffeine: What Can You Believe?...............65

Chapter 16: Pass the Salt? Or Pass Up the Salt?...........68

Chapter 17: Carbohydrates: Why Spaghetti
  Is OK On Your Diet.................................71
Chapter 18: How's Your HDL Level?.......................74
Chapter 19: The Great Vitamin C Debate..................77
Chapter 20: The Mysterious Case of Vitamin E...........80
Chapter 21: Dieting: There's No Shortcut...............83
Chapter 22: Are There People Who Can't
  Lose Weight?......................................86
Ideal Weights..89
Section III - Substance Abuse..........................91
Chapter 23: Warning: The Surgeon General Is Right......93
Chapter 24: Quitting Cigarettes: You Can Do It.........96
Chapter 25: An Alcoholic? Me?!.........................99
Chapter 26: Living With an Alcoholic..................102
Chapter 27: Marijuana—Is It Really the Safe Drug?.....105
Chapter 28: Cocaine: The Flight to Nowhere............108
Section IV - Major Diseases...........................111
Chapter 29: How to Give Your Heart
  a Fighting Chance.................................112
Chapter 30: After a Heart Attack—Life Goes On.........115
Chapter 31: Is It the Big "C"?........................118
Chapter 32: Cancer: What We Know
  About Prevention..................................121
Chapter 33: What's Your B.P.?.........................124
Chapter 34: Diabetes: Living Without Sugar............127
Chapter 35: The Holiday Blues.........................130
Section V - Stress....................................133
Chapter 36: Are You a "Type A"?.......................134
Chapter 37: How to Hypnotize Yourself.................137

Chapter 38: When You Can't Sleep................................141

Chapter 39: Maybe It Really <u>Is</u> the Best Medicine.........144

Section VI - The "Little" Things...............................147

Chapter 40: Fever: The Body's Germ Killer..................148

Chapter 41: Backache: Is It Inevitable?.......................151

Chapter 42: Are You That One In Ten?.......................154

Chapter 43: Is It Safe to Sun?...................................157

Chapter 44: Eyes—Only Two to a Customer.................160

Chapter 45: Look Ma—No Cavities!...........................163

Section VII - The Medical Profession........................166

Chapter 46: Choosing and Using a Doctor: A Quiz.......167

Chapter 47: The Annual Physical:
  Too Much of a Good Thing?..................................170

Chapter 48: Your Health, Your Responsibility.............173

Acknowledgments

I am grateful to Alison Walker for tireless research assistance, and to Dr. Thomas Coates, Associate Professor of Medicine and Co-director of the Behavioral Medicine Unit of the School of Medicine, University of California at San Francisco, for technical consultation and review of this book.

A lot of my knowledge of the health and fitness movement comes from my involvement in "Live For Life", the employee health program at Johnson & Johnson. I am grateful to everyone who pioneered that program, from Chairman of the Board Jim Burke on down.

Several friends, relatives, and co-workers suggested subjects for this book; they have my gratitude.

Finally, I would be remiss if I did not pay homage to a writer whose reputation among medical professionals is at least as high as the esteem of her readers. More than any other writer, Jane Brody of *The New York Times* has spread the gospel about health and fitness. Her books, columns, and articles have inspired and enlightened me, and I thank her.

Kenneth H. Franklin
Fairfield, New Jersey

Foreword

We're in the middle of a health revolution.

The evidence is everywhere. It's in the language—people are talking about "fiber" and "resting pulse rates" the way they used to talk about the latest TV show. It's on the streets—you have to watch where you walk these days for fear of being knocked flat by a passing jogger or cyclist. And it's in the doctors' offices—where people are coming to ask for help in *preventing* disease, rather than waiting until they come down with something and then expecting the doctor to cure it.

Once, people looked upon health as something for the doctor to worry about. Most of the time they didn't think about health—until they lost it. Now, people want to know how to *stay* healthy. They have read about nutrition, and exercise, and stress, and how to live longer with less risk of serious disease, and they like the idea.

What about you? You're probably a busy executive, important to your company, with a lot on your mind besides your health. Your main job *is* your job. If you have time, you may try to squeeze in a visit to the health club, and you've been meaning to talk to your spouse about cutting back on fattening dinners. But somehow, the health revolution may have gone on without you.

And yet, you're well aware of what's at stake. Perhaps one of your friends or someone at work has had a serious heart attack, or cancer. Maybe *you* have a health problem yourself. You know you should be doing something to cut your risk and make yourself feel better. But what, exactly, should you do?

That's why we wrote this book. We wanted to create a catalog of lifestyle improvements, something busy executives could read through at their leisure. You can skim around from one section to another. If you see something that appeals to you, give it a try. If something else isn't right for you, forget it. Health, in spite of what you may think, is not an all-or-nothing proposition. If someone tells you to exercise *and* lose weight, and all you want to do for now is exercise, that's fine!

What will this book do for you? Well, it *won't* show you how to run a 26-mile marathon, or give you recipes for Tibetan bean curd, or chastise you for having a drink before dinner. Instead, our hope is that it will show you how simple it is to make a few worthwhile changes in your life—changes that can honestly make a big difference in how you feel, how long you live—and how well you do your job.

In writing this book, we've tried to avoid treating you as either a complete idiot who knows nothing about how to take care of yourself, or as a granola-and-tofu fanatic who lives for the opportunity to deny himself yet another earthly pleasure. We all know that health is important, but so are other things—your job, your family, your plans for the future. Good health is the best way to ensure you'll be able to enjoy all of those important things in your life.

You see, we—the people who created this book—live in the same world you do. We're business people, just like you. We've studied the health and fitness field for years, and we've learned a lot about what's important. But we've never gotten so swept up by the enthusiasm of the health movement that we've lost our perspective.

The ideas we've come up with here are ideas you can make a part of your life without changing so much that the people in the office will look at you funny. What we're really after is substituting some common-sense health habits for other habits—which may be common, but lack good sense—that somehow or other got stuck in place before you knew better.

Now you *do* know better. That's why you're reading this book. You may not feel like joining any revolution just yet, but you want to make a start toward improving your health and fitness, and keeping it that way. We congratulate you.

Here's to your health!

Section I - Exercise

"You gotta try jogging! You can really work up a good sweat!"

"Tennis? That's too tame for me! If you've never played racquetball, you don't know what you're missing!"

"What? You play golf? Don't you know that's not exercise?"

I'm afraid that some of my fellow fitness adherents tend to turn people off when they talk like this. If you've ever been at the receiving end of this kind of verbal coercion, please try to restrain your hostile impulses, and keep an open mind. Exercise, believe it or not, really is both good for you and fun.

As we say in Chapter 1, the blame for much of the world's antipathy to exercise can be laid on our childhood and military experience. When I was growing up in the fifties and sixties, exercise was either a form of punishment or something that people in authority, like parents or drill sergeants, made us do because it was good for us. Sort of like spinach, or going to bed before the good TV shows start.

Man—by which I mean men and women—was meant to move. Unlike such creatures as the hippopotamus and the slug, man was given long, articulated legs, and arms capable of wondrous feats of mobility. When we sit at our oaken thrones and conduct our executive business, taking time out only to go to lunch and go to the bathroom, we do not do our bodies any favor. The human body, as we have begun to learn, is a prime illustration of the maxim, "Use it or lose it."

In short, when we don't use our bodies, we risk losing them to a host of ailments that nobody wants to even think about.

But I don't want you to get the idea that exercise's only value is to prevent disease. It really can be fun! What's more, exercise can help you feel better, look better, and work better. If you don't believe *me*, ask that jogger in the next office. If we can just get over our life-long prejudices —in fact, if we could just come up with some other word besides "exercise"—we might be able to see things positively. Maybe if we made it illegal, and said it would ruin your health, we could start a run on running. Who knows?

At any rate, my purpose in this section is to give you some ideas that may make it easier to start your own body in motion. Read with an open mind. Throw out those images of army calisthenics and gym class humiliations.

Why You Hate Exercise (And What to Do About It)

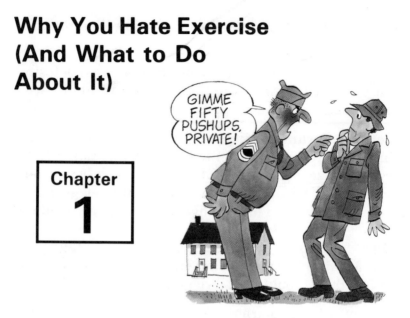

Chapter 1

The way we were brought up to think about exercise, it's a wonder __anyone__ enjoys it.

It's a pity they call exercise "exercise". The word has all sorts of unpleasant associations for most of us. A much better word would be "fun".

What happened? How did we get to the point where anything that makes us use our muscles and get a little out of breath is awful? How come the thought of fitness gives us a cold shudder and sends us to the refrigerator for something tasty to calm us down?

Consider our childhood. What do all kids like to do? Run around. What do all parents tell their kids to stop doing? Running around.

We go to school. We take gym. We are exposed to

organized sports. Organized—that's where they take all the fun out of everything and give you a grade, so you know whether you liked it or not. And anytime they don't have an organized sport for you to "play", they get you doing—yuck!—calisthenics. Some kids liked gym. They were called "jocks". Everyone else hated it, and anything connected with exercise.

Gym class wasn't the only time you were exposed to organized forms of exercise. There's the military. "Awright, you sorry-looking recruits," growls the drill sergeant, "I wanna see 50 push-ups, and then 50 sit-ups, and then 10 laps around the field. Or else!"

At least he doesn't ask you to enjoy it.

When we grow up being told that physical activity is something we shouldn't do, or something we have to organize, or something just for "jocks" and "health nuts", or something we *will* do or else—it's little wonder that so many adults confine their exercise to lifting their forks and bending their elbows.

Kids have the right idea. There's nothing more natural than playing. It's how every animal in the world stays in shape. It's only when we take the fun out of it that we lose interest.

What we should be doing is encouraging our kids to do whatever playing they enjoy (within reason, of course). Do they like to run around? Great! That's something they can do all their lives, and there are few better ways of staying fit and healthy.

For us adults, it's a question of realizing how we got this negative attitude about exercise in the first place, and then proving to ourselves that it can still be fun.

What we do is less important than that we do *something*. There are exercises that are better than others. But the best exercise in the world is no good unless it's fun. If you don't enjoy it, you probably won't do it for long. Find something you enjoy, like walking, gardening, running, racquetball, or whatever. Find some other person or people to do it with. Don't push yourself to unrealistic goals. And reward yourself for your efforts—make it a reward that is special for *you*. Some people find that the way they feel after a good workout is all the reward they need!

The Best Thing Since Sliced Bread

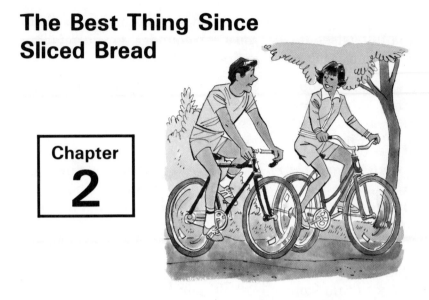

<table>
<tr><td>Chapter

2</td></tr>
</table>

The benefits of exercise—every day the list gets longer.

Everyone knows that exercise is good for you. But *why* it's good is less understood. Even the people who are already exercising probably don't realize all the good things they're doing, so we're going to give you a quick rundown of the most important ones.

First, we should define what we mean by exercise. We're talking about aerobic exercise, the kind that gets you moving vigorously enough to speed up your heartbeat for at least 20 minutes at a time, at least three times a week.

Immediate Benefits

• *Relieves tension.* Feeling depressed, uptight, or angry? A good workout gets rid of your stress—and does a better job of it than a cigarette or a double martini.

- *Improves sleep.* Not only does vigorous exercise help you fall asleep faster, you sleep sounder, so you get more good from each hour you're asleep.

- *Reduces appetite.* Really! Many people think it's the other way around, but exercise is actually an appetite depressant. That's one reason it's best to exercise before meals, rather than after.

- *Stimulates the mind.* When you go for a three-mile jog or brisk walk, your mind tends to wander. When your mind wanders, it often comes up with surprisingly brilliant thoughts.

- *Promotes companionship.* A lot of people are doing all sorts of exercise these days. If you exercise, you're likely to find someone who'll join you.

- *It's fun.* If the exercise you choose is something you like to do, you're more likely to stick with it. And the more you do it, the more fun it will be.

Long-Term Benefits

- *Strengthens the heart.* The more you exercise, the more blood your heart can pump with each beat. So it doesn't have to beat as often, which is good.

- *Improves circulation.* As you exercise, your body actually develops additional capillaries—the tiny blood vessels that deliver oxygen to the cells. The more capillaries, the more oxygen gets to the cells, which is also good.

- *Controls weight.* Besides reducing appetite, exercise increases metabolism, which helps you burn more calories even when you're not exercising.

- *Increases HDL.* HDL is a kind of protein in the blood that scientists have found helps remove harmful build-ups of cholesterol in the blood vessels. People who exercise have more HDL than inactive people do. (See Chapter 18 for more on HDL.)

- *Eases hypertension.* People who get regular aerobic exercise have lower blood pressure than people who don't. And people who have high blood pressure can bring it down by exercising. (Check with the doctor first.)

- *Helps treat diabetes.* Exercise increases a person's sensitivity to insulin. For diabetics, this means more effective treatment of their disease with less need for insulin.

- *Strengthens bones.* A leading cause of disability among people over 50 is fractures caused by gradually weakening bones. Exercise helps keep bones strong.

- *Trims the figure.* Where there may have been fat, exercise creates muscles. Where there may have been unwanted bulges and unflattering flabbiness, exercise brings sleek, lean, firm profiles.

- *Makes you feel alive.* There's nothing like a good stiff workout to make you feel alert and alive. And it's a feeling that lasts long after you've stopped sweating.

How Much Exercise Is Enough?

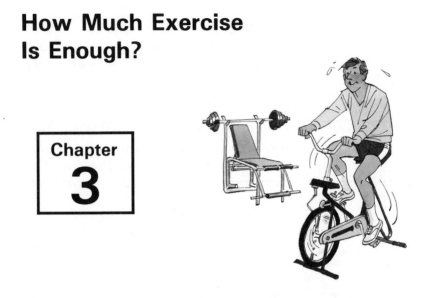

Chapter

3

One hour per week may be enough—but there are a few ground rules.

If you thought that the only way to get your body in shape was to take up residence in the nearest gym, we've got some good news for you. Fitness—and we're talking about the kind of fitness that strengthens your heart—takes surprisingly little time to achieve and maintain.

One hour a week should do it. But that doesn't mean one hour all at one time; that's probably worse than *no* exercise since it puts your system through stresses and strains that it's not prepared for. Spread the hour over three 20-minute sessions, with a day or two of rest in between each.

Here are some guidelines that will help you get the most out of your workouts:

1. Not just any exercise will make you fit. Sports like bowling, baseball, golf, and even football—which are all characterized by short bursts of movement followed by periods of inactivity—are great for fun and recreation. But for fitness you need something that will keep you moving for at least *20 minutes at a time*. Some activities that do that are listed in the chart on page 38.

2. Do you hate running? Then running is obviously not your exercise. Find something you like. Better yet, find something you and a friend like. The more support you get from others, the more you'll enjoy yourself. If you don't enjoy your exercise, the prospect of better fitness at some indefinite time in the future will not be enough to get you to stay with it three times a week. It has to be fun.

3. Take five minutes before you start and five minutes after you finish to warm up and cool down. Muscles—especially your heart—don't like sudden changes. If you step up the pace gradually you'll lessen the jolt to the system. What you're after is *training*, not straining.

4. If you're also trying to lose weight, vigorous exercise will help. In addition to the calories you burn up while you're exercising, there is a carry-over effect. For up to 15 hours after you stop, your body continues to burn more calories than normal. Of course, you can't lose as much weight with exercise alone as you can by combining it with a reduced-calorie diet.

5. If you're out of shape, or have any medical condition, or if you're over 40—check with the doctor first. It may be unnecessary, but do it just to be safe. Tell him or her what you plan to do, and ask if you need a checkup first. Chances are, the good doctor will congratulate you on your good sense!

Exercise Palaces: Welcome to the Club!

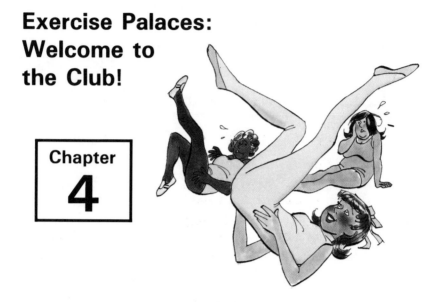

Chapter

4

Some clubs are into health. Others are just into your wallet.

For some people, membership in a health club is the perfect way to exercise and lose weight without having to go it alone. One of the clubs' biggest assets is the prospect of meeting people who share your interest in slimming down and firming up, people whose encouragement might keep you going on days when you'd rather curl up in front of the TV.

That's not all, of course. Some clubs hire highly skilled exercise counselors who can tailor an exercise program to your individual needs and help you achieve specific goals. And some health club members are happy just having a place to work out where they can stay warm and dry.

The New York Times says that ten new health clubs

open every year in the borough of Manhattan alone. The International Racquet Sports Association puts the amount spent by the average health club member each year at close to $500. The health club industry is said to be taking in well over $5 billion a year. Clearly, some people are making a lot of money from America's renewed interest in staying fit.

In an ideal world, this would all be to the good. What better use for one's money than one's health, you might ask. Many, perhaps most, of the thousands of health clubs throughout the country are operated competently and honestly, and their members have trimmer profiles, firmer muscles, and healthier hearts to show for the money they spend there. But other clubs are just out to make a quick buck. Too often the people who sign up at these places lose not only their money, but their interest in exercise as well.

Some guidelines for choosing the right club for you:

• *Never join a club that you haven't seen.* Some ads glowingly describe clubs that are "due to open soon" and offer special rates if you sign up in advance. No matter how attractive those rates sound, don't bite. The files of Better Business Bureaus from coast to coast are full of complaints from sadder-but-wiser would-be health clubbers who paid their money to clubs that never opened. Even if the club does open, you have no way of knowing how well you'll like it if you haven't seen it first.

• *Check it out at the time you'll use it.* If you plan on doing all your workouts at 10 a.m. or 3 p.m. you probably won't have much trouble with crowds. But if your work schedule forces you to fit your exercising into the early

23

morning, lunchtime, early evening, or anytime on weekends, things can get a bit tight at many clubs. Some are geared for the crush, but others aren't—there just aren't enough Nautilus machines or racquetball courts or showers to go around. The only way to find out before you join is to take a tour of the facility at the time you're most likely to use it.

• *Talk to members.* Ask the people you see working out how they like the club. (But don't let the club choose the people you talk to.)

• *Read the contract carefully.* If you have to move out of the area before your membership expires, can you get a partial refund? Or transfer your membership to another club? If you change your mind a day or two after you sign up, can you back out of the deal? (In some states, the law requires this kind of cooling-off period.)

• *What does the fee include?* Will you have to pay extra for towels, exercise classes, lockers, etc.? Are there budget plans that might apply to you? Make sure your membership isn't going to become so expensive that you never use the club.

• *Is this the right club for you?* Before you join, make sure the club you're considering has the features you're looking for. Some clubs emphasize racquet sports, some offer an array of exercise machines, some are aimed at swimmers, and others have everything. But some health clubs are primarily reducing salons, with "exercise" limited to sitting in a steam room or undergoing a massage. If you're after aerobic exercise, you need something a little more strenuous than passive sweating.

Running—the Fad That Never Faded

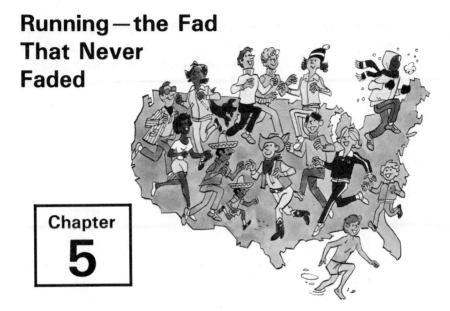

It's become a national pastime.

In spite of the way some people carry on, running (also called jogging) is not the only exercise worth the effort. Running is just one of a number of aerobic conditioning exercises (see chart, page 38). Running is not even the best of these, according to some experts. Runners face a higher risk of injury to joints and muscles than walkers, swimmers, or bikers, for example.

Nevertheless, running is enormously popular. When the sport bloomed in the late 70's some called it a fad—but it never faded away. Today, some estimates place the number of Americans who run fairly regularly at nearly 40 million. In almost every city and town in America, the sight of joggers is so common that people hardly notice them anymore. Running has become part of the American scene.

Why *is* running so popular? Probably the main reason is that it's easy—at least in the sense that you don't need any special skills or expensive equipment to do it. Everyone older than two knows how to run. Unlike some sports and exercises, running is something you can do virtually anywhere, anytime. You can run with a friend, with a crowd, or by yourself. You can run to lose weight, run to get or stay in shape, run to win races, or just run for fun. You can run a couple of miles every couple of days, or you can run 20 miles every day. In short, you can run almost any way you like, and you'll still get the benefits.

Those benefits are the same as for any other good aerobic exercise—a healthier heart, lower blood pressure, an easier time controlling weight, and improved feeling of self-worth. You also build up muscle tone in your lower body. (But not much in your upper body, which is one reason to supplement your running with weight-lifting, swimming, or some other above-the-waist exercise.)

Let's say you've never run farther than from the car to the house during a pouring rain, but now you'd like to give jogging a try. There are some simple steps you ought to take to make sure that running is a pleasant—and life-long—experience. Here's how to get started:

1. *Make sure you're in condition.* If you're older than 40, check with your doctor before beginning any exercise program. At any age, check with the doctor if you're significantly overweight, or you have high blood pressure, or any other condition that places restrictions on your ability to exercise.

2. *Get some good shoes.* Running shoes are the only equipment you need to run. Don't skimp. Go to a store

that sells many brands, and try them on. Pick the one that feels right for you. You may have to spend up to $50 or more, but it will be money well spent.

3. *Start slower than you think you have to.* If you're a beginner, don't expect to start out running five-mile races the first week. Start with slow jogging, alternating with walking. Don't run to the point of exhaustion. The idea is to gradually build your endurance. The idea is *not* to push yourself to unrealistic limits.

4. *Stretch.* As we said before, running poses a higher risk of injury than some other exercises. The best way to cut down the risk is to stretch your muscles before *and after* running. See page 40 for some good runners' stretches.

5. *Make it fun.* More runners quit running out of boredom than for any other reason. But it doesn't have to be boring; in Chapter 6 we'll discuss some ways to make running not just bearable, but actually interesting. Even fun!

The More It's Fun, the More You'll Run

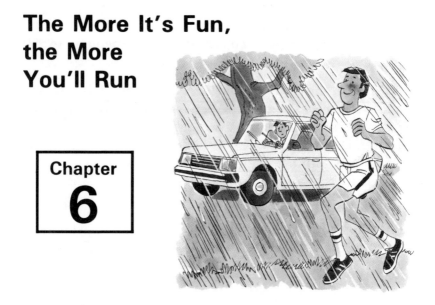

Chapter

6

Running is boring only if you don't use your imagination now and then.

Anyone who runs is bound to encounter people who say things like, "Running? Isn't that incredibly boring?" It can be, of course, but it certainly doesn't have to be. Regular runners have come up with a number of ideas that help keep their running from becoming a chore. Maybe some of them will work for you.

• *Add variety.* A lot of runners who quit out of boredom run only around tracks or on treadmills. Of course that's boring—but that's not where you should be running. Get out on the roads and trails, and make up different routes each time you run. Next time you take a business trip, bring your running clothes and explore the area while you run—you'll see things you'd miss in a car. If you normally run through city streets, try some unpaved country roads for a change. Or skip the roads entirely, and run through a park or a forest, or along a lake, or anywhere the terrain is friendly and there's no problem with trespassing. Another change you can try: Go out for a run in the middle of the night, when you have the world to yourself. (Use common sense about where you do late-night running, of course.)

• *Chart your progress.* You'll get a nice feeling of accomplishment when you run farther or faster than you have before. A lot of runners like to chart their improving capability by keeping a logbook, where they jot down the miles and time of each run, as well as anything special they want to remember. There's something very satisfying about looking back to the early days and realizing how far you've come. This doesn't mean that you have to be competitive about all your runs, though. And business people who live highly competitive lives at the office should allow their running to provide a break from all that.

• *Allow yourself to gloat.* If you become a runner, you're doing something that most people haven't been able, for one reason or another, to handle—you're taking care of your own health and fitness. If that notion causes you to feel superior to the overweight, underexercised people you pass during your runs, why shouldn't you? (Some runners find it especially satisfying to go for runs in the rain, or when it's very cold, and they glory in the looks of puzzlement they get.)

• *Try a race or two.* The important thing to keep in mind about running races is, you're not in them to win. You're in them to beat your own personal record, or to enjoy the companionship of other runners, or just to get yourself a fancy tee shirt. Whatever your objective, races are one of the ways of making the sport more fun.

• *Run when you feel low.* You don't have to restrict your running to times you feel great. It's an excellent cure for a host of head problems—such as tension, anger, grief, boredom, anxiety, fear, and even hunger. Next time you've got troubles, instead of washing them away with alcohol or food, try sweating them off with your feet.

• *Use your runs for daydreaming.* Critics who say running is boring cite the fact that you have nothing to do with your mind as their proof. But the other side of that argument is that some of your most creative thinking occurs when there are no distractions—like when you're all alone and running. You'd be surprised at how many office crises you can solve during a vigorous five-mile run.

• *Watch for once-in-a-lifetime runs.* Some runs you never forget. It could be on a tropical beach you have all to yourself early some morning. Maybe it will be an encounter with a family of deer during a run through the woods. It may even be the thrill of finishing your first marathon. That kind of experience makes all the sweat and sore muscles worthwhile.

Walking—It's Better Than You Think

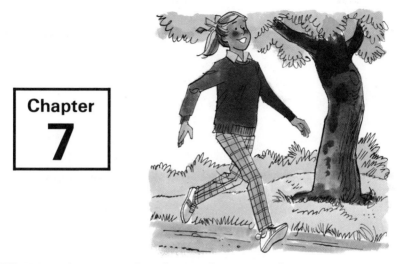

Walking just may be the perfect exercise.

Mention the word exercise to some people, and they immediately conjure up images of gasping, sweating, and exhaustion. To the committed, all those things are fine—the sweat and tired muscles are part of the fun of exercise. But strenuous exercise isn't appealing to everyone.

If you're not into sweat, walking could be for you. It may not *seem* like exercise—everyone does it, and there's no special skill involved—but those are really two of the reasons why walking is right for almost anyone.

There are different ways of walking, and different degrees of benefit you can derive. A casual stroll around the block won't do much for your aerobic fitness, although it sure beats sitting in front of the TV. More beneficial, though, is something a little faster-paced and longer-lasting. While everyone has different capacities and different goals, many experts recommend you work up to a brisk walk of three miles or so, which should take about an hour. If you get three or four of these walks in every week, that should be all you need to get in shape.

Walking is deceptive. Since it's so easy, it's hard to believe that it could be that good for you. But walking is almost as good a conditioner as running. It will burn up just as many calories per mile—about 125. It strengthens the heart, lowers blood pressure and resting pulse rate, increases muscle tone, and relieves stress. It's a good way of getting from where you are to where you're going. And it's a great way to get out and see the things that you miss when you're driving past them at 40 miles an hour.

Walking is something everyone knows how to do. You don't need any special equipment, other than a good pair of shoes (running shoes are best). Unlike running and other strenuous activities, walking poses almost no risk of injury. And walking is convenient—you can walk anywhere, anytime, alone or with a crowd.

You say walking isn't convenient for you? Try these ideas:

• When you have a short errand to do, walk instead of driving.

• Walk to work. If it's too far, park half a mile from work and walk the rest of the way.

• Walk to the person's desk instead of using the phone.

• In bad weather, do your walking at an indoor shopping mall.

• Get a friend to walk with you. It's more fun that way . . . and the friend will thank you!

Of course, you don't have to start out doing three miles, or going at a three-mile-per-hour clip. Start with what you feel comfortable doing for now. Increase the pace and distance when you feel you're ready.

Next time someone tells you to take a walk, thank them—and do it!

Cycling: One Wheel or Two?

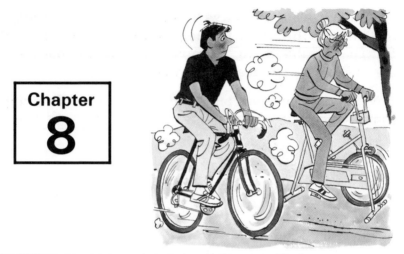

Whether you cycle indoors or out, it's still an excellent way of shaping up.

It's a good thing most kids learn to ride a bike when they're young. If they waited until they were older, they'd probably find out that it's used for exercise, and never go near the thing.

Sure, riding a bicycle is good for you—but that doesn't take any of the fun out of it. The fact that you'll probably enjoy bike-riding makes it one of the best exercises you can do. If other physical conditioning regimens leave you bored or exhausted, the two-wheeler in your basement may be just what you're looking for. Some good reasons:

• Like running, bike-riding is an excellent way to strengthen your heart, lower blood pressure, and work off calories.

- Unlike running, riding a bike is unlikely to cause problems with the feet, ankles, and knees.

- Bicycles, if you've forgotten, are a good way to get where you're going—in fact, about a half-million Americans ride their bikes to work.

- Cycling is something you can do alone, or with your family, or with a whole crowd of other riders.

- A bicycle gives you the opportunity to see the countryside you miss while driving a car.

In recent years, there has been a rise in the popularity of a variation on the bicycle—the exercise bike. Selling for anywhere between $50 and $500 or more, this one-wheel mutation combines the muscle-building advantages of a standard bicycle with the convenience of working out at home.

Of course, the big drawback of exercycling is that it can be boring. After all, you don't see much scenery. But there are ways of holding the drudgery to a minimum. Try reading while you work out. Some exercycle manufacturers sell stands that hold a book or magazine in front of you. These stands can be bolted right to the bike.

Or you can just watch TV or listen to music—difficult or impossible while riding a regular bicycle, but no problem if you work out at home. Certainly a lot better for you than watching TV from your easy chair!

If the bike you ride is the kind with one wheel, there aren't many safety precautions to worry about—just do a little slow, easy pedaling before and after your workout. But if you're going to be riding the roads, keep these tips in mind:

1. *Obey all traffic rules.* Ride on the right, watch out for pedestrians, signal for turns, and use lights and reflectors for riding after sunset.

2. *Keep your bike working properly.* Make sure moving parts are lubricated, nuts and bolts are tight, and tires are fully inflated.

3. *Watch out for road hazards.* The biggest hazard of all is cars—some will watch out for *you*, others won't even see you. Assume that you might have to get out of their way. Also beware of potholes, sewer gratings, patches of ice, and sand or gravel. All can cause you to lose control if you're not careful.

4. *Protect yourself.* Many bicycle riders wear helmets, some with attached rearview mirrors—for spotting those cars. A jacket or long-sleeved shirt is also a good idea.

5. *Know how to handle your bike.* The place to learn how to use a brand new ten-speed isn't on the busiest street in town—ideally, it's in an empty parking lot. This is a particularly important point if your kids get a new bike: Make sure they know how to handle it under all conditions before you turn them loose on the roads.

Whether your bicycle takes you across the country or nowhere at all, it's a great way to get the Number One muscle—your heart—in shape.

Which Exercises Are Best?

All exercise is helpful, to some extent. But if you're trying to increase your general fitness, strengthen your heart, and boost your endurance level, some exercises are better suited than others. The best cardiovascular exercises are those that get your heart rate up to what is called the "target zone" and keep it there for at least 20 minutes at a time. A minimum of three times a week—or every other day—is required. More often is even better.

To find your "target zone", first subtract your age from 220. That will give you your *maximum* heart rate. The target zone—the range at which heart conditioning takes place—is between 70 and 85 percent of that figure. For example, if you are 45 years old, your maximum heart rate is 175 (220 - 45 = 175), and your target zone is 123 to 149. Thus, any exercise that speeds up your pulse to between 123 and 149 beats per minute for 20 minutes or more is an effective cardiovascular conditioner.

To measure your pulse, gently place your index and middle finger in the crevasse at the side of your neck, just below your jaw. If you can't feel a pulse there, try just below the base of the thumb, on the side of the wrist. Once you locate the pulse, all you have to do is count the beats.

The best procedure for measuring exercise pulse rate is to check the pulse for 10 seconds immediately after you stop the exercise (it's too difficult to get an accurate reading while you're still moving around), and then multiply by six. The result will be your pulse in beats per minute.

On these pages, we list some common types of physical activity, both recreational and non-recreational, ranging from sitting quietly to strenuous exercises. The column for calorie use gives an approximate figure for the exercise as performed for 20 minutes by a person weighing 150 pounds. If you weight more, you'll burn more; if you weigh less, you'll burn less. The figures don't include a nice little bonus—people who exercise burn more calories even when they're not exercising. In any case, if you're trying to bring your weight down, you need to burn up 3,500 calories to lose one pound of fat. Obviously, if you cut your calorie intake at the same time you increase your exercise level, the job will be easier.

Activity	Calories	Benefits
Quiet sitting	25	Outside of relaxation, none.
Slow walking	60	Enjoy the scenery. No exercise value for most people.
Bowling	80	Some muscle-building value—for one arm. No cardiovascular benefit.
Golf (power cart)	100	Not continuous or strenuous enough. Better: no cart.
Moderate walking	100	Some conditioning value for people with low capacity. A good starter exercise.
Slow swimming	100	Fair all-around, moderate exercise. But not vigorous enough to strengthen the heart.
Housework (e.g., vacuuming, washing floors, raking leaves)	80-150	The harder, the better. If you keep going, without a rest for 20 minutes or more, you're really exercising.

Brisk walking	150	Very good, safe, invigorating exercise. At three to four miles per hour, walking is a heart-builder.
Tennis	100-160	The key is to play hard, without a break. Singles is best, but a hard-fought doubles match is good too.
Fast swimming	175	Swimming laps in a pool, without stopping for a rest, is an excellent cardiovascular exercise.
Bicycling	80-250	At low speeds, you get some muscle building in lower body; at high speeds, sustained for 20 minutes or more, you also get excellent heart and lung conditioning.
Aerobics/ calisthenics	150-250	If there's steady, rhythmic movement, these can be excellent conditioners.
Skiing	150-300	Downhill is fun, but not much help in building fitness. Cross-country skiing, though, is one of the best there is. Very demanding.
Handball, racquet-ball, paddleball, or squash	200-300	As long as the game is fast, evenly-matched, and continuous, any of these can be great conditioners.
Jogging/running	200-400	Millions swear by it, and they're right. A superb way to build endurance and heart-lung capacity.

Before the Run—
Stretching Those Muscles

Some people perform stretching exercises to develop muscle strength, but most stretching is done as a preliminary to other exercises, to improve flexibility and to prevent injury. The way stretching protects muscles is by warming them up, and by lengthening them. A warm, long muscle is less likely to tear or strain when subjected to the stresses of prolonged exercise.

The stretches shown here are designed primarily to be done before running, but it's a good idea to stretch before any exercise. You don't necessarily have to limit yourself to these stretches; for example, see Chapter 41 for some stretches to help the back. If your exercise involves using the upper body, you should stretch those areas as well.

A couple of rules for stretching:

1. Slow, gentle, smooth stretching is the right way. The wrong way is fast, vigorous bouncing. That can tear the muscles you're trying to protect.

2. When you start to stretch, go only as far as is comfortable—you're not looking for pain. After holding that position for about 15 seconds, relax for a moment. Then repeat, trying to go a little further into the stretch. If you can't go further without pain, don't. No purpose is served by subjecting your muscles to more than they can take.

3. While you're stretching, breathe normally. Don't hold your breath.

FOR THE BACK OF THE THIGHS

1. Bend at the waist to a 90-degree angle, so your back is parallel to the ground.

2. Extend your arms straight out and grab something secure, like a countertop or a tree branch.

3. Slowly push your back down toward the ground, but don't let go with your hands.

4. Hold for about 15 seconds, relax, then repeat.

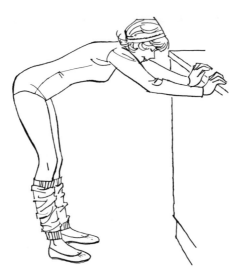

FOR THE BACK OF THE CALVES

1. Stand a few feet away from a vertical support, such as a wall or tree.

2. Extend your arms to the support, keep your back straight and your feet flat on the ground, and gradually lean your body toward the support.

3. Lean only until you feel the muscles stretch. Hold for 15 seconds, relax, then repeat.

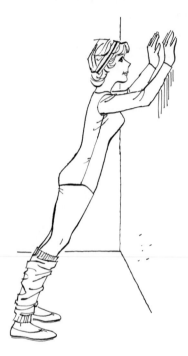

FOR THE FRONT OF THE THIGHS

1. Hold onto a secure support, such as the one you used in the first stretch.

2. Bend one leg at the knee, grab the ankle, and gently pull up, toward the buttocks.

3. Pull only until you feel the stretch, hold for 15 seconds, then change legs. Repeat.

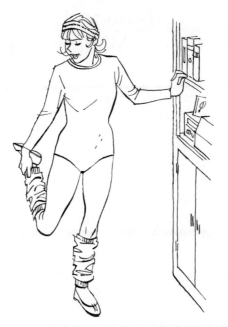

FOR THE INSIDE OF THE THIGHS

1. Squat down with one leg bent and the other out to the side, as straight as is comfortable. Support yourself with your hands on the ground.

2. Hold for 15 seconds, then change legs. Repeat.

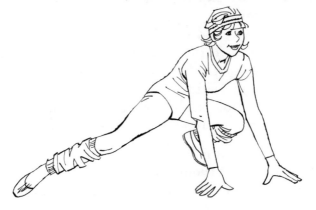

Section II
Nutrition & Weight Control

I read an interesting interview the other day. The fellow being interviewed was one of the pioneers of the health and fitness movement. To the question, "How do you know what to eat and what not to eat?" he replied, "If man made it, I don't eat it."

That's a little extreme (although the advice has kept this man, now in his late sixties, in top shape). I'm a believer in moderation. I think it's unrealistic to expect people to give up all the foods they've learned to enjoy over the years. It's hard to make a convincing case that an occasional candy bar, jelly donut, or serving of french fries will do anyone any lasting harm. It's when these kinds of foods become the mainstay of a diet that it's time to make some changes.

In this section, we'll talk about some of the dietary changes that seem to have the biggest potential for improving your well-being, both short- and long-term. We'll talk about vitamins, we'll talk about fiber, we'll talk about carbohydrates. We'll show you how to eat snacks that are actually good for you. We'll urge you to think about some new ideas for breakfast, and we'll caution you about the dangers of salt, cholesterol, and caffeine. We'll guide you through a salad bar, pointing out the items that aren't really in the health-food category. And we'll give you some help if you're trying to lose weight.

It all adds up to a case for moderation. We've tried to avoid the kind of textbook-sounding advice a lot of nutrition writers fall prey to. "No more red meat!" they warn.

"Shun sugar! Forswear fats! Abandon all alcohol, and fill up on fiber!"

People who talk like that don't live in the same world the rest of us inhabit. The concept of healthful living doesn't require the total and permanent exclusion of everything that's fun in life. Just keep a few guidelines in mind, and leave the self-denial to the monks.

Food—the Good Guys and the Bad Guys

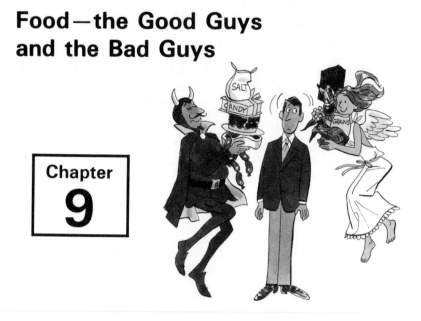

Chapter 9

What's good to eat? What's bad?
Here are some helpful guidelines.

"Eat more vegetables."

"Eat less fried food."

"Increase your protein intake."

"Watch out for cholesterol."

"Cut down on carbohydrates."

Confused? It almost seems as though that's what they want—all the people who keep telling us what the ideal diet should consist of. It's little wonder that some people just give up trying to follow the rules, and go ahead and eat what they feel like.

We hope we don't add to your confusion, but we've got some more rules. But take heart—these rules are easy to understand, they're not controversial, and they cover just about everything you need to know, in general, about the foods you should and should not eat. They're also approved by the National Institutes of Health and by most medical groups.

Rule Number One: Eat a variety of foods. Fad diets that restrict you to all protein, or no carbohydrates, or any other unbalanced regimen cause you to miss out on important nutrients that even a vitamin pill can't replace. You should include foods from all four food groups every day—fruits and vegetables; breads and cereals; dairy products; and meat, poultry, fish, and beans.

Rule Number Two: Eat to maintain your ideal weight. If you don't know your ideal weight, ask your doctor or check the chart on page 89. If you're overweight, you can lose pounds by reducing your calorie intake— gradually is best—and by increasing your exercise, also gradually. Keep in mind that it takes 3,500 calories to make a pound of body fat. If you want to lose ten pounds, you can do it in less than ten weeks by just cutting out one piece of pastry a day and exercising three times a week for a half hour. Once you're at your proper weight, don't stop your good habits! (See Chapter 21.)

Rule Number Three: Limit fats, especially saturated fat, and cholesterol. Americans get too much saturated fat in their diets, mostly from meat. Some fat is necessary, but more of it should come from polyunsaturated fats, the kind you get from vegetables and vegetable oils. Cholesterol is found in most of the same foods as saturated fat, as well as eggs and some shellfish. You don't have to stop eating these things—just use moderation. (See Chapter 18.)

Rule Number Four: Eat foods high in starch and fiber. There are several good reasons for choosing foods that supply starch (carbohydrates) and fiber: (1) Most of these foods also contain a wide variety of vitamins and minerals; (2) most of these foods are relatively low in calories; and (3) fiber is good for the digestive system in many ways. The foods to look for are fruits, vegetables, whole grain cereals and bread, and nuts. (See Chapter 12.)

Rule Number Five: Avoid too much sugar. Foods high in sugar are also apt to be (1) high in calories, (2) low in nutrition, and (3) high in cost. Sugar causes or contributes to tooth decay, overweight, diabetes, and possibly heart disease. Instead of eating something sugary like cake, cookies, or candy, why not choose something like a piece of fruit or some popcorn?

Rule Number Six: Avoid too much sodium. In effect, this means avoiding too much salt, the major source of sodium in our foods. One way to cut back is to use the salt shaker a little more sparingly at the table. But a lot of processed foods have salt in them, so you should read labels carefully. Why avoid sodium? Doctors think it may contribute to high blood pressure, a major cause of heart disease. There's also recent evidence that sodium makes people more sensitive to the harmful effects of stress. (See Chapter 16.)

Rule Number Seven: Use alcohol in moderation. A glass or two of wine or beer with dinner may help digestion and relieve stress. But too much alcohol, besides leading to alcoholism, is linked to heart disease, cancer, liver disease, and traffic accidents, to name a few potential dangers.

All seven of these rules are important. But if you forget everything else, try at least to remember the first rule— eat a variety of foods. That's the best way to make sure you get enough of what you need and avoid too much of what you don't want.

Pizza for Breakfast?

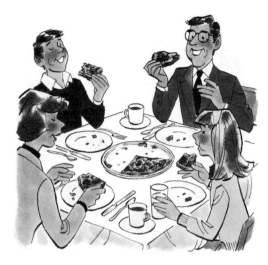

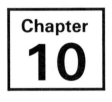

Maybe you don't eat breakfast because you don't like the menu.

There was a time when families ate breakfast together —even on weekdays. The meal may have consisted of eggs, bacon, toast, juice, coffee, and perhaps a piece of fruit. Or maybe it was just a bowl of oatmeal. Or, on Sunday, the menu may have featured waffles or pancakes, and ham or sausage.

Nowadays, the family breakfast is an endangered species. No one seems to have time to sit down a half hour in the morning—there's too much of a rush getting to school or work. Some people still manage to gulp down a bowl of whatever ready-to-eat cereal is around, while others make do with a quick cup of coffee and a Danish. Or if they're really rushed, people may gobble down a "breakfast bar"—which is not much different nutritionally from an ordinary candy bar.

But even these people are doing better than the millions who skip breakfast entirely. Why do they do it? A lot of people just don't have any appetite in the morning. And others, trying to lose weight, figure that eliminating that first meal is an easy way to cut calories.

That's a mistake. Study after study has shown that dieters who don't eat breakfast frequently lose less weight than those who eat three meals a day. Apparently, what they eat during the rest of the day more than makes up for the breakfast calories they miss.

Another reason many people shun breakfast is that they just don't like traditional breakfast food. Maybe it's the thought of soggy corn flakes or runny eggs that puts them off. Or perhaps they're worried about the nitrites and cholesterol in bacon, or the sugar in ready-to-eat cereals, or the fat in everything from a cheese omelette to the cream in their coffee.

But who's to say that traditional breakfast foods are the only things we can have in the morning? There is absolutely nothing in our biological makeup that makes tuna fish salad, or even leftover pizza, for example, a nutritious lunch but not good for us as breakfast. If you find breakfast less than exciting, or you want to make some nutritional improvements, try something new for a change. Tomorrow morning, how about—

—*Reheated leftovers.* Did you have spaghetti for dinner last night? It takes less time to reheat the leftovers than to fry an egg and bacon. And it's better for you— eggs and bacon are loaded with cholesterol. Spaghetti isn't.

—*A sandwich.* We know, it sounds weird. Sandwiches

are for lunch. But your stomach can't tell time. What's sound nutrition at noon is just as sound at 7 a.m.

—*Soup*. Another food that sounds like lunch, but is easy to fix and a good source of balanced nutrients.

If you can, try to get a variety—from one day to another, and in each breakfast. Our bodies need protein, fats, and carbohydrates, as well as fiber and all those vitamins and minerals. The best way to be sure of getting them is by having several kinds of food at each meal.

Mom was right—eat your breakfast!

Snacks That Are Good for You

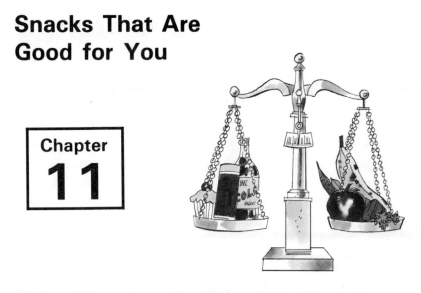

Chapter 11

We've all heard you shouldn't eat between meals—especially on a diet. But if eat you must, there are healthful ways to do it.

It's three-fifteen in the afternoon. Lunch was over a couple of hours ago. You notice a gnawing at your stomach. You begin to think about having something to quiet the hunger pangs. A candy bar? A can of soda? A piece of pastry? Everything sounds delicious.

Stop for a minute. Whether you're trying to lose weight or not, you know that those goodies are just empty calories—no nutrition. Deep down you know your doctor would be annoyed with you for eating stuff like that. And your dentist would too. But you're hungry! What can you do?

Believe it or not, there are plenty of snacks that are good for you *and* taste good. Some suggestions:

• *Cold and wet:* Instead of a can of soda pop (which is mainly water, sugar, and flavoring), how about a glass of orange juice? As the ads say, "It isn't just for breakfast anymore." If not OJ, any other fruit juice is great too. If you can't get juice, try iced tea or iced coffee—without sugar (you can teach yourself to like it that way).

• *Munchies:* Forget about that candy bar, or that cupcake, or that bag of potato chips. How long since you had a cool, crisp apple? How about a juicy fresh navel orange? Want something more chewy? Carrots are hard to beat. Something you don't have to keep in the refrigerator? Bananas.

Some fruit is just as sweet as candy, but it's not empty calories. You get a whole bunch of vitamins, minerals, and fiber in the bargain. The problem is, many of us grew up thinking of fruits and vegetables as something we *had* to eat or our parents wouldn't let us have dessert. Dessert, usually one of those high-calorie goodies, became a way of rewarding ourselves. Fruit and vegetables were the cost, the penalty, the bad medicine we had to endure to get our reward.

Too bad, really. All those things nature grows for us are actually delicious. Give it a try—bring an apple to work tomorrow. Skip that trip to the candy machine just once. It's not a big deal. It's a little thing—a nice little favor you can do for your health.

Does this mean you'll never again be able to enjoy the pleasures of Twinkies and ice-cream cones? Of course not. Make those things an occasional treat. Just don't forget the "occasional" part.

P.S.: Of all the traditional snack foods you can eat, one

stands out as clearly better for you than the others. Surprise—it's popcorn! Lots less calories (leave off the butter), less fats and grease, less sugar (almost none) than the rest. If you have to have something from the snack machine, make it popcorn.

What's So Good About Fiber?

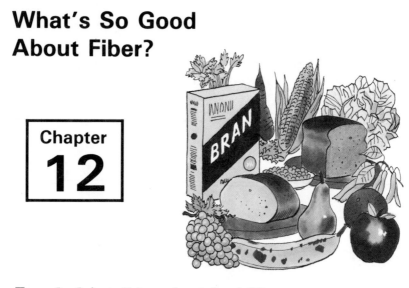

Chapter
12

Everybody's talking about food fiber.
Is it just another fad?

Well, not to leave you in suspense any longer, the answer is no. Fiber is *not* just another fad. Scientists don't know everything about food fiber yet, but they do know enough to be able to tell us we should be getting more of it than most of us now do.

Fiber comes in several varieties, and its role is to help the body digest other foods. Fiber comes only from plants —you won't get any fiber from a steak or scrambled eggs. Fiber is what your grandmother used to call "roughage".

And as your grandmother knew, fiber is good for you. Here are some of the things the experts have found fiber does:

- Lowers the cholesterol in your blood

- Helps diabetics control their blood sugar level

- Reduces blood pressure

- Prevents gallstones

- Makes it easier to cut back on calories

- Alleviates a host of intestinal problems, including constipation, spastic colon, diverticulosis, and possibly cancer of the colon.

Some doctors have likened fiber's effect on the body to that of a magnet—picking up harmful substances like fats and chemicals, and holding on to them until they can be eliminated. Besides harmful substances, fiber also soaks up water—that explains why it can help dieters. When fibrous foods get into your stomach, they sponge up water, swell up, and give you a full feeling—before you can eat too many calories.

So how do you get fiber?

As we said, it comes only in plants. Just about any vegetable, any fruit, any grain has at least some fiber. You've probably heard that bran is a good source—it's one of the best. But many doctors feel that the fiber in fresh or frozen fruits and vegetables is better—more effective at doing what fiber does, and easier on your system.

Some specific foods:

- Breakfast cereals—all the bran cereals, plus shredded wheat and Grape Nuts.

- Whole-grain foods—whole wheat bread, rye bread, brown rice.

- Vegetables—carrots, peas, celery, cabbage, potatoes,

corn, beans. (Served raw where possible, or cooked *al dente*—excessive cooking destroys the fiber.)

- Fruits—apples, pears, bananas, oranges, grapes.

How much fiber do you need?

Again, the evidence is not all in. As with any food, the amount you need probably depends on what else you're eating, how good your general health is, and your body's own workings. If you're not getting much fiber now, you should increase your intake gradually. If you have any medical conditions that restrict your diet, you ought to talk to your doctor before adding a lot of fiber. And don't forget to eat a balanced diet—fiber is just one part.

Beyond those words of caution, there's not much harm you can do by eating as much fiber as you want. Good old roughage—it turns out that grandmother was right all along.

Salad Bars: What to Pick

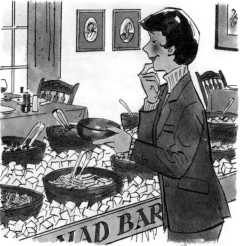

Beware! Not everything in the salad bar is low-calorie health food.

It's sort of ironic—people go to a restaurant so they can enjoy being waited on, and then what do they do? They head for the salad bar, where they wait on themselves. And the number of people who are fixing their own salads grows every day. The salad bar is seen in everything from fast-food outlets to posh white-linen restaurants.

It isn't hard to see the reason for this phenomenon. People are more interested in their health and fitness these days, and salad is perceived as a healthful food. If you're on a diet, the salad bar may seem like the safest place to have a nutritious meal while avoiding excessive calories.

In general, that's true. But there are traps. A lot of what shows up at many salad bars is loaded with calories, short on nutrients, or both. To separate the goodies from the not-so-goodies, here's a guided tour through a typical salad bar:

First stop: *the lettuce*. It's the foundation of any salad, so of course you'll want to have some. All leafy greens are low in calories, but how nutritious are they? Iceberg lettuce, the one usually served, is also the lowest in vitamins and minerals of all lettuces. Better alternatives are Romaine lettuce, chicory, or spinach leaves.

Raw vegetables. Relatively new to people's concepts of what belongs in a salad are a few vegetables that used to be served only cooked—broccoli, cauliflower, mushrooms. Here's one place to load up your plate. Broccoli is an excellent source of vitamins and fiber. Cauliflower and mushrooms aren't quite as rich in vitamins, but virtually all vegetables at the salad bar are good sources of fiber, and are low in calories.

Traditional salad ingredients. Tomatoes, onions, green peppers, carrots, cucumbers, radishes—these are what most people think of as the stuff you mix with your lettuce to get a tasty and colorful tossed salad. They're all fine— low in calories, high in fiber, and, in varying degrees, good sources of vitamins A and C. If you're looking for something to eat a lot of without ruining your diet, cucumbers are hard to beat—you could eat three *pounds* of cukes and still wind up with fewer calories than are in a glass of beer. As for onions, they may not make a big hit when you get back to the office, but some studies show they can actually help reduce the risk of heart disease.

Pickles and olives. Use with care. Relatively low in calories, but not especially rich in vitamins. And loaded with something you don't need in your salad bowl: salt. Salt is suspected of contributing to high blood pressure in millions of people.

Mayonnaise salads. Cole slaw, potato salad, and macaroni salad—do we really have to tell you? Mayonnaise is loaded with calories and cholesterol. If you want to have a *little* of these, and your diet can afford it, cole slaw is the best nutritional bargain of the three. It's made with cabbage, a good source of vitamin C. Another creamy dish to go easy on is cottage cheese. In spite of the widely-held perception to the contrary, cottage cheese is *not* diet food. It's a pretty good source of protein, but at the cost of calories, salt, and cholesterol.

Antipasto. Some of the more elaborate salad bars have things like ham, salami, and several kinds of cheese. A little won't hurt you. But they're not health food. High in fat, high in sodium, high in calories. If you load up with these things, you'd probably have been better off ordering from the menu.

Dressings. Most prepared salad dressings are high in calories, and should be used in moderation. All of them— even diet dressing—are high in salt. Best bet: a little oil and vinegar. No salt at all.

So what's the answer: Should you choose the salad bar? Yes, by all means. Even with the nutritional no-no's you may encounter, it still offers excellent variety. And if your diet has variety, chances are that at least some of it is good for you.

Is **Fast** Food the Same As **Junk** Food?

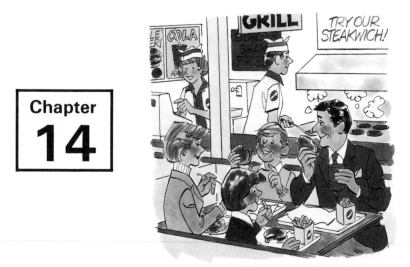

Surprise—you can get a reasonably nutritious meal at a burger palace.

The last place you'd expect to find "health food" would be a fast-food restaurant. While they've become a significant part of our national eating habits, no one goes to McDonald's, Arby's, or Pizza Hut in search of vitamins. But the food served in these restaurants is far from being "junk" food. With a little care, you can get a reasonably nutritious meal.

Take hamburgers, for example. A regular burger at most of the chains would have about 250 calories, and would be about 25 percent protein, 25 percent fat, and 50 percent carbohydrates. That's roughly the ratio recommended by nutritionists. You'd get about 17 percent of your daily protein requirement from the burger, along with lesser amounts of some B-complex vitamins and some minerals.

Or french fries—hardly most people's idea of a healthful food. But potatoes are a good source of vitamin C, and you even get modest amounts of some other vitamins.

Suppose you chose pizza. Nothing to feel guilty about there—pizza is more nutritionally balanced than a lot of soups and sandwiches. All that cheese gives you calcium and vitamin D, the tomato sauce adds vitamin A, and you also get plenty of protein, iron, and B-complex vitamins. The calories are roughly comparable to other fast-food items.

Not that you have to limit yourself to these choices. Some places are going farther than the burger-and-fries route, and offering salad bars. Even if you just use the salad bar to add lettuce and tomato to your cheeseburger it's a plus. (See Chapter 13.)

All of which adds up to this: There's nothing wrong with an occasional visit to the burger, chicken, fish, roast beef, or pizza palace of your choice. It's when those visits become less occasional and more regular that the nutritional shortcomings begin to matter.

A lot of working people eat a significant portion of their meals at fast-food restaurants. Unless they're eating at a salad bar, they're probably shortchanging themselves of several important vitamins and minerals. There's also a real risk of getting too much sodium (salt), and too many calories. A meal of a large hamburger, order of fries, and a shake can easily add up to more than half of some people's daily recommended calorie intake. It's OK for most people, occasionally. But it's *not* OK for anyone *all* the time, especially for anyone on a calorie-counting diet or for people who need to restrict their sodium intake.

If you find yourself pulling up to these eateries more than a couple of times a week, here are a few ways to increase your nutritional batting average:

• Choose the restaurants that let you make it your way. If you can add your own fixings to a hamburger, the lettuce, tomato, and onion you put on will contribute fiber and vitamins. If you ask them to leave off the pickle and ketchup, you reduce the sodium significantly.

• Watch what you drink. Most people order a soft drink, but all you get in soda pop is sugar, caffeine, and water. Even a shake is better—it's not a *milk* shake (it's made with vegetable oil), but it contains some protein, calcium, and B vitamins. Better choices: milk, or fruit juice.

• If you're ordering fried chicken, skin the bird. Most of the fat is in the skin. If you peel it off, you'll be left with a relatively low-fat, low-calorie, high-protein meal.

• Make sure your other meals make up the difference. As we said, there's nothing wrong with an occasional fast-food meal. Just be sure that you get whatever nutrition that meal lacks somewhere else. Like at your own dinner table, for example.

Caffeine: What Can You Believe?

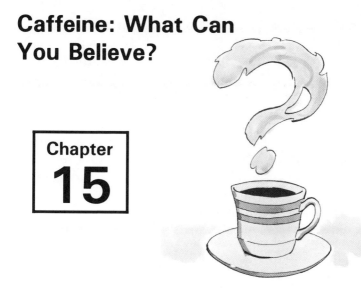

If all the controversy about caffeine has you confused, you're not alone.

If you listen to all those advertisements for caffeine-free beverages, you may start to believe caffeine is the number-one health threat in the country. In spite of the fact that more than 10,000 articles and reports have analyzed every possible link between caffeine and its effect on the human body, there is still no consensus among doctors and scientists about this substance.

At least there's no *definite* consensus. But what seems to be emerging is a general feeling that perhaps we've overstated the dangers of caffeine a bit. Some very respected researchers are willing to go on record that caffeine is OK, except for some people, and provided it's not overdone.

Caffeine, as most people know, is the stuff in coffee that

gives you the lift that gets you started in the morning and gets you through the day. Caffeine is a drug, a chemical that has the power to stimulate the mind and produce several physiological changes in the body. It takes about five minutes after consumption before caffeine has spread throughout the entire body.

Of course, you don't have to drink coffee to get caffeine into your bloodstream. There's almost as much caffeine in tea, and soft drinks are another major source. Chocolate and cocoa have caffeine, as do some common over-the-counter medicines, such as pain relievers and diet pills.

Some—perhaps most—of the changes that caffeine causes are beneficial. Besides being a pick-me-up, caffeine helps you think more clearly, relieves drowsiness, heightens the senses of smell and taste, shortens reaction time, and gives an overall sense of well-being. It's no exaggeration to say that many people do their best work with a cup of coffee at their side.

But at what cost? What about all the reports linking caffeine with such problems as heart disease, cancer of the breast, bladder, and pancreas, and birth defects? This is the reason we still lack a consensus—some studies indicate there *is* a cause-and-effect relationship, and others say there isn't.

About all that can be said at this point is that every time someone has published a report linking caffeine to a particular health problem, other scientists have been unable to confirm the findings. Often the initial study turns out to have had flaws in procedure, casting doubt on the validity of its warnings. This doesn't mean that caffeine has been proven totally safe, but it does mean that no one has yet proved it definitely harmful.

On the other hand, common sense tells you that caffeine should be avoided right before bedtime. Even if that cup of coffee or tea doesn't keep you awake (and it might), it does interfere with normal sleep patterns. Whatever sleep you get won't do you as much good as if you hadn't had the caffeine.

There are people who should use caffeine with caution, or not at all. They include pregnant women (because caffeine taken in by the mother gets into the unborn baby's blood, and there's still some question about the consequent risks to the baby's health), people with a history of heart problems (because high doses of caffeine can cause irregular heartbeat in some people), and anyone else whose doctor recommends a limit on caffeine consumption. Children get most of their caffeine from soda; as long as they don't overdo it most don't get enough to worry about.

Of course, *no one* should overdo caffeine. Caffeine is a drug, and overuse can lead to a mild form of addiction, which causes all sorts of problems anytime you can't have your cup of coffee. Too much caffeine has also been related to headaches, stomach pains, and diarrhea.

But used in moderation, caffeine seems to be as safe a stimulant as we've got. "Caffeine has been part of our society for a thousand years," says one scientist, "and it's probably the most socially accepted drug we've got. I doubt that it's going to go away." Adds another: "Save your willpower for the things that matter."

Pass the Salt?
Or Pass Up
the Salt?

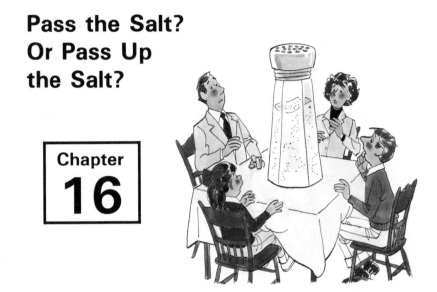

Chapter
16

In recent years there has been a growing volume of articles in almost every newspaper and magazine in the country about the hazards of salt. We're told what will happen to us if we eat too much salt, and we're given a list of foods that are high in salt. The list includes such obviously salty items as potato chips and pretzels, soy sauce and anchovies, sauerkraut and pickles. But it also includes, we learn to our dismay, such foods as cottage cheese, tomato sauce, and canned tuna. (Actually, these foods aren't necessarily salty—they may just be high in sodium. Salt is made up of sodium and chloride, but sodium is part of many other compounds as well.)

It's really not surprising that a lot of people get discouraged. It almost looks as though they'll have to give up everything they like in order to get their salt intake down to recommended levels.

But don't despair. In the first place, there are many

people who really don't have to spend a lot of time worrying about salt at all. Unless you have high blood pressure, or your doctor says you're likely to develop it in the future, the best course to follow is moderation. And don't forget the other guidelines for nutritious eating.

If you *do* have high blood pressure, or if close relatives do, your doctor may suggest that you restrict your salt intake. If so, you're wise to follow that advice. High blood pressure is one of the major causes of heart attacks and strokes. And the sodium in salt is almost certainly a major cause of high blood pressure.

Here are a few ideas that may help if you want to cut back:

• *Cut down gradually.* Humans at birth don't need salt to enjoy their food—it's a taste they have to learn. A taste for unsalty food can be learned too, but it takes time. Start by reducing the amount of salt you add to food in cooking and at the table. After a while, cut back some more. Where possible, switch to low-salt versions of foods. If you take it gradually, you won't miss the salt at all.

• *Taste first.* Are you in the habit of sprinkling salt on everything you eat, without tasting first? It's a good habit to break. You'll be surprised to find that a lot of things taste fine without adding any salt.

• *Use a substitute.* There are commercially available salt substitutes you can buy; most of these are made by replacing sodium with potassium. If you don't want to use one of these, try this homemade mixture: Combine two tablespoons of dry mustard powder with one tablespoon each of onion powder (not onion salt), dried lemon peel, dried crushed basil, and dried crushed thyme. Put the mixture in your salt shaker and use it the way you'd use salt.

• *Avoid processed foods.* With rare exceptions, things like TV dinners, canned vegetables, and snack foods are made with a lot of salt. The more you can cut back on these items the less salt you'll get. And watch out for fast-food restaurants. Most of the things they sell are high in sodium.

• *Read labels.* You won't always know you're eating something high in salt or sodium unless you check the label. Watch out for anything that has sodium in it—such as monosodium glutamate (MSG) or even baking soda.

We still have a lot to learn about the effects of salt and sodium. Recent studies point to a relationship between salt and sensitivity to stress, and some scientists believe everyone should cut back drastically on salt intake. Others say salt isn't the villain it's being portrayed. In cases like this, where the experts can't agree, the best bet is to err on the side of caution. There's no way you can get too *little* sodium.

Pass the salt, please, but just a sprinkle.

Carbohydrates: Why Spaghetti Is OK On Your Diet

Chapter
17

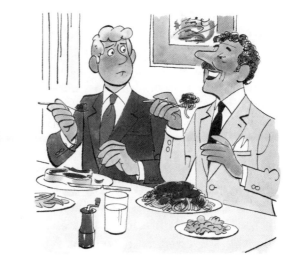

*If it grows in the ground, and it's food,
it's probably good for you.*

Carbohydrates are probably the most misunderstood nutritional subject around, and certainly one of the most controversial. On one side, there is a group led by Dr. Robert Atkins swearing that carbohydrates are the cause of a variety of diseases and disorders, and we ought to eliminate them from our diet. And on the other are people like Nathan Pritikin who urge us to significantly increase our intake of carbohydrates and eliminate just about everything else.

As is so often the case in matters of nutrition, the path preferred by most experts lies somewhere between the two extremes. But that path is closer to the high-carbohydrate Pritikin regimen than it is to Dr. Atkins' diet. The fact is, most Americans need more carbohydrates in their diet.

What are carbohydrates? They're one of the three basic nutritional elements, the others being fats and protein. Carbohydrates are found in almost every food that comes from the farm. Vegetables and fruits are among the best sources, as are grains and cereals and the foods made from them, like bread and pasta.

Another abundant source of carbohydrates is sugar, and that raises a confusing point about this subject. While many doctors urge us to eat more carbohydrates, they're really talking about *complex* carbohydrates. *Simple* carbohydrates are the sugars, and we already get more than we should of those. Complex carbohydrates are the starches, and they're found in the foods we are told to eat more of. In other words, the message is to eat more carbohydrates, but only the complex kind.

The reason many experts don't completely buy the Pritikin approach—drastic reduction of fats and protein —is that we need a balanced intake of all three food elements. A diet that severely limits a whole group of foods with nutritional value deprives the body of vitamins and minerals that it might not be able to get anywhere else. That's why most quick weight-loss fad diets are unhealthy, and why most experts advise a policy of nutritional moderation.

We still haven't said anything about *why* carbohydrates are so great. Here's a partial list:

• Carbohydrates supply energy. The body can burn

almost anything it eats to get energy, but the most efficient source is carbohydrates.

• Carbohydrate foods contain fiber. Fiber is another substance Americans need more of, and the place to find fiber is the same place as carbohydrates: fruits, vegetables, whole grains, cereals, bread, and pasta. (See Chapter 12.)

• Carbohydrates help you lose weight. Hard to believe that potatoes, bread, and spaghetti are better "diet" foods than steak and cottage cheese, but it's true. Excess body fat is burned most completely in the presence of carbohydrates, and foods high in complex carbohydrates fill you up with fewer calories than foods high in fats or sugar.

• Carbohydrates help protect against disease. According to a study by the Federal government, countries whose populations have the lowest incidence of heart disease are also the ones whose people eat the most carbohydrates. Southern Italians, for example, eat very little fats but lots of carbohydrates in the form of bread and pasta. Their blood is much lower in artery-clogging cholesterol than that of northern Europeans who eat more meat.

While all of these reasons are important, people who eat zucchini and rice and bran muffins and noodles and apples don't care that much about the scientific rationale for their food. They just eat that stuff because it tastes good!

How's Your HDL Level?

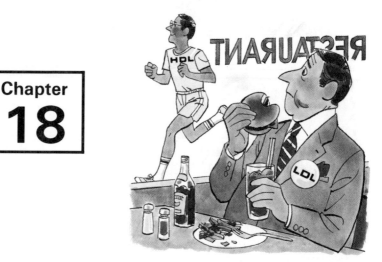

Chapter 18

Not all cholesterol is bad for you. HDL to the rescue!

Cholesterol is one of those topics that have been covered so extensively in the media by now that some people automatically tune out as soon as they hear the word. Of course, there's a reason for all the attention in the press—and anyone concerned about health and fitness ought to listen.

For years, cholesterol was suspected of playing an important part in heart disease. But until recently, hard evidence about the cause-and-effect relationship was lacking. In 1984, however, a decade-long study by the National Heart, Lung and Blood Institute took the question mark away. Cholesterol, the study concluded, *is* a major cause of heart attacks, and lowering the amount of cholesterol in the blood lowers the heart attack risk significantly.

The problem of too much cholesterol is widespread, especially in the United States. While there are several factors involved in determining the level of blood cholesterol, the most important is probably diet. Foods that are high in cholesterol and saturated fat both contribute to the problem. Most of the foods in that category come from animals—red meats, eggs, and dairy products are among the prime examples. In other words, the foods that Americans love most.

But there's more to this story. Not all cholesterol is the same. There are components called low-density lipoproteins and high-density lipoproteins. LDLs and HDLs. LDLs are the bad guys. They're the part of cholesterol that brings fatty deposits to every part of the body, including the blood vessels, and leaves it there.

HDLs, on the other hand, apparently try to undo the harm that LDLs do. They circulate throughout the body, pick up fatty deposits, and remove them from the blood.

Naturally, the question becomes: How do I get more HDLs and fewer LDLs? Answer: There are several ways. Among the most effective:

1. Substitute polyunsaturated fat for saturated fat. What that entails in practice is eating less steak and hamburger, and more fish and chicken. Less butter and more margarine. Less whole milk and more skim milk. Fewer eggs, or at least fewer egg *yolks*.

2. Eat more fiber. Foods that are high in fiber tend to lower the LDL level. Fiber is in most fruits and vegetables, and whole-grain bread and cereals.

3. Exercise. If you get regular (at least three times a week), sustained (at least 20 minutes at a time, without

resting), vigorous (hard enough to raise your pulse to about 140 beats per minute) exercise, you can significantly raise your HDL level.

It's easy to tell people what to do, but how many of us are ready to abandon the joys of our favorite foods for the vague promise of better arterial health? Cholesterol reduction, like any other healthful lifestyle change, is a matter of doing the best you can in ways that are the easiest for you.

For some people, the most important factors are beyond their control. There are people who are genetically programmed for high levels of LDL cholesterol, and almost nothing can change that. And there are other fortunate individuals who can indulge in ham and eggs to their hearts' content. For some reason, their bodies are more efficient at keeping their LDL level low and the HDLs high.

For the rest of us, the best protection comes from following the rules. It's a life-long proposition. But the payoff is big—a little less worry about the Number One killer, heart attack.

The Great Vitamin C Debate

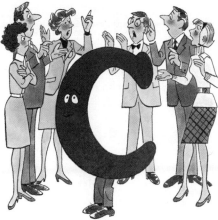

Vitamin C prevents scurvy. They're still arguing about what else it does.

To hear some people tell it, vitamin C can prevent or cure everything from the common cold to cancer. On the other side are people who are equally convinced that vitamin C is the subject of a giant rip-off of consumers too ready to believe the substance has magical powers.

What's the truth?

To put it simply, we still don't know. Or at least we don't know for sure. But new information is coming to light every day about this hotly debated nutrient.

Vitamin C, or ascorbic acid, is one of the group of essential substances that human beings can't manufacture in their bodies, and so have to take regularly either in food or in pills. Since vitamin C is water soluble, it is constantly being lost along with the water the body loses. So you have to take vitamin C every day.

The Government says you need 60 milligrams of vitamin C daily to prevent scurvy. That's about the amount in a glass of orange juice. But many people take a lot more than that. Linus Pauling, for one, recommends up to *10,000* milligrams a day. But Dr. Pauling claims vitamin C does a lot more than prevent scurvy.

Among the claims made for vitamin C, taken in large doses:

• It prevents colds, or makes them less severe, or reduces their duration.

• It prevents some kinds of cancer, and cures others.

• It lowers the amount of cholesterol in the blood.

• It treats such psychiatric disorders as schizophrenia, depression, and senility.

• It can lessen the severity of arthritis, diabetes, and some forms of bone disease.

Mind you, these claims aren't yet universally accepted as true. Far from it. But *some* scientists are finding that some of these assertions may be valid. It's pretty certain, for example, that vitamin C protects against the cancer-causing effect of nitrosamines, which are products of the nitrites in some meats, such as bacon. A few years ago, the government began requiring that all bacon that contains nitrites also contain vitamin C.

With a lot of uncertainty still clouding the truth about vitamin C, it's hard to know what course to follow.

Doctors are divided on the subject. Some feel there's relatively little risk involved in taking large doses of the vitamin, so many people do it just to be safe. Others are waiting to find out the results of current research.

If you decide to increase your vitamin C dosage beyond what you get in your food, you may want to check with your doctor first, to make sure he or she isn't aware of any reason you shouldn't. And when you go shopping for the vitamin, be forewarned: It's very easy to spend a lot more than you have to. Vitamin C comes in sizes all the way from 100 milligrams up to 1,500 milligrams per pill. You can get "rose hips" vitamin C, vitamin C with bio-flavonoids, all-natural vitamin C, and so on. But all vitamin C is essentially the same, and the best procedure is just to find the best price you can.

Vitamin C—probably not the cure-all its partisans claim, but also probably a lot more than just a way to keep from getting scurvy.

The Mysterious Case of Vitamin E

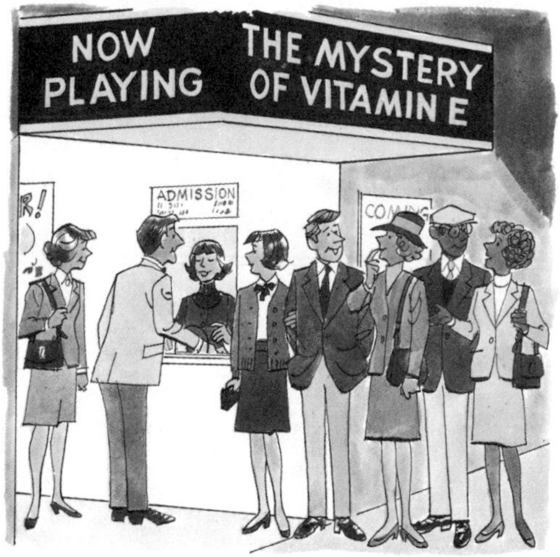

Chapter

20

Vitamin E is still a mystery, but we're starting to unravel it.

Vitamin E was once called "the vitamin in search of a disease". Today, more than 60 years after its discovery, scientists are still puzzled over the vitamin's true role in human nutrition. A lot of questions about vitamin E remain to be answered. But some of the facts are beginning to emerge:

Q.: How much vitamin E should people take?

A.: The government-established daily requirement is 30 International Units, but research has so far failed to demonstrate any symptoms of vitamin E deficiency. Thus, unlike other vitamins, vitamin E *appears* not to be essential to human health.

Q.: *Then why should I take vitamin E?*

A.: For two reasons: First, deficiency of vitamin E in laboratory animals *does* bring about serious health problems, so it's only prudent to assume problems are possible in at least some people. And second, vitamin E appears to have some potent beneficial effects.

Q.: *Such as?*

A.: Some studies suggest that larger-than-normal doses of vitamin E may protect the lungs against damage from nitrogen dioxide and ozone, two chemical air pollutants. In addition, the vitamin blocks the formation of cancer-causing nitrosamines, which are produced in the body from the nitrites used as preservatives in some foods. Vitamin E is also useful as a treatment for non-cancerous cysts in the breast, a disorder that affects up to 20 percent of American women.

Q.: *Is there any danger from taking large doses of vitamin E?*

A.: If the vitamin builds up in your body it can cause hives or rashes. If that happens, just lay off vitamin E for a while. Also, the vitamin enhances the action of anticoagulant medicine, and the combination can cause internal bleeding. Otherwise, though, the vitamin doesn't have any known toxic effects.

Q.: *What about the theory that vitamin E can slow down the aging process?*

A.: That's still being studied. Results of some animal tests indicate that vitamin E's antioxidant properties may slow down the deterioration of body cells—which is partly a process of oxidation. No one has proved that what happens under carefully arranged laboratory conditions will happen in people. But a lot of vitamin researchers are taking a daily vitamin E supplement, just in case.

Q.: And those rumors that vitamin E is the "sex vitamin"—any truth?

A.: The best answer to this is that anything that makes people *think* they have increased sexual powers probably has a positive effect. The fact that there is no known scientific basis for it isn't that important.

Q.: What are the best sources of vitamin E?

A.: Vegetable oils, margarine, wheat germ, whole-grain cereals and bread, liver, Brussels sprouts, green leafy vegetables, and soybeans. Or you can take a vitamin pill if you want more than you're getting from your food. It can't do any harm, and it might do a lot of good.

Dieting: There's No Shortcut

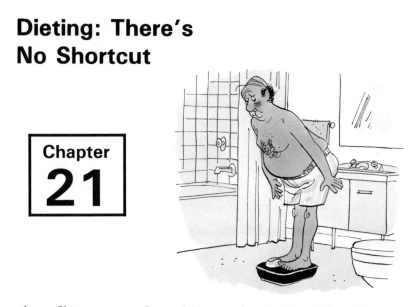

Chapter

21

Any diet can work—while you're on it. After that, though, the pounds come back.

Those glowing testimonials for the latest miracle diet plan sure sound convincing. "I lost 10 pounds in 14 days!" "I went from a size 12 to a 7 in just three weeks!" "I melted the inches off in no time!" And so on.

Whether based on pills, starvation, or some strict diet regimen like grapefruit or eggs, these plans all have one thing in common: They work only while you're on the diet. No matter how successful you are at losing weight during the diet itself, the odds are overwhelming that you'll put it right back on when you go back to your normal eating habits. (Some diet plans aren't even good for you while you're on them. Because they limit you to specific foods, you may not be getting the nutrition you need.)

There's only one reason people weigh more than they should: They're taking in more calories than they're using up. And there are just two ways to solve that problem: Take in fewer calories, or use up more. Or better yet, do both. But that means *all* the time—not just for a few weeks while you're slimming down. And as far as the calorie input end of things is concerned, that means changing your eating habits.

Changing the way you eat requires willpower, determination, patience, and a good bit of common sense. But it can be done. Here are some tips that can make it easier for you:

• The main idea is to *eat a variety of good wholesome foods you like*, but eat *smaller portions* of them. Most diets ultimately fail because they try to force you to eat things you aren't going to be happy with for long.

• *Don't skip meals.* It's unhealthy, and you'll probably end up eating more calories in the meals you do eat than you'd save by skipping one. Remember, you're trying to form new eating habits, and three meals a day is one of the habits you should include.

• Along with your reduced portions, you should *increase your exercise*. In addition to the extra calories you'll burn off, exercise actually reduces your appetite.

• *Drink plenty of water.* It fills you up, it has no calories, it's good for you, it's free—what more could you ask!

• *Eat slowly.* You'll feel full faster.

• *Easy on the sauces, gravies, and toppings.* A serving of some green vegetable is only a few calories, but a tablespoon of butter or margarine on top adds 100 more.

- *Avoid "empty" calories*—things you eat or drink that provide little or no nutrition. Things like candy, pastry, soda, and alcoholic beverages.

- Try this trick: *Use a smaller plate for dinner.* You'll fill it up with less food, but you won't feel you're getting cheated as much as if you put the small portion on a big plate.

- *Don't go food shopping when you're hungry.* You'll buy things you don't really need.

- *Stay away from the refrigerator between meals.* One of the best new habits you can form is to confine your eating to three times a day.

- If you're trying to lose a lot of weight—more than 10 or 20 pounds—it might be easier to *do it in stages.* After you've lost 10 pounds or so, take a breather, maintain the loss, and start losing again when you're ready. Even a moderate weight loss is helpful.

- One more trick: When the going gets tough, just concentrate on how you're going to look after all those pounds have gone away. It'll give you the strength to keep going—try it!

Are There People Who Can't Lose Weight?

"I have a gland problem."

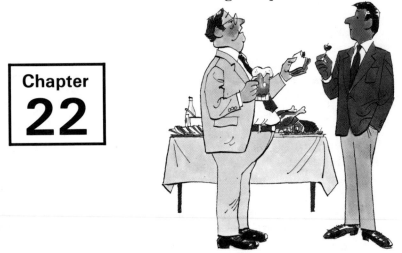

Some people are convinced that no diet will work for them.

There are as many reasons why people put on too much weight as there are ways of taking it off. For some people it's as simple as an inability to resist anything made out of chocolate. For others, the culprit is too many bottles of beer. But for many, overweight is tied to a deep-seated personality characteristic that causes them to eat compulsively as a substitute for other forms of gratification that they're unable to achieve.

When food has become a substitute for love, or control, or success, cutting down on eating is not a simple matter of saying no to dessert. Nor is the answer to be found in a fad diet of any kind. Doctors say that some people who overeat are just as addicted as if their excessive behavior were related to drugs or alcohol. And, surprisingly, the treatment for food junkies is very similar to the treatment for alcoholics and drug addicts.

As with those problems, the first step in coming to grips with compulsive eating is to recognize that you *have* a problem. Have you tried to lose weight—perhaps several times—with either no success at all or success at first, followed by a speedy return of the unwanted pounds? Have you stubbornly stayed on strict diets for weeks or months, and been frustrated by your inability to reach your goal? Do you find yourself heading to the refrigerator anytime something upsetting happens? And do you find yourself coming up with all sorts of rationalizations for your weight problem? Some of the most common excuses: "No matter how much I diet I can't lose weight," "It's only temporary—I'll start a diet right after_____," "It's _____'s fault for making me cook big meals and buy fattening food," and especially this one: "I have a gland problem."

A few—very few—people *do* have a thyroid gland problem that can affect their weight. More likely than a deficient thyroid, though, is an addiction to food. When you come right down to it, eating more calories than you burn up is the only cause of overweight. The fat comes from somewhere—you don't absorb it from the air. People who swear that no matter how little they eat they can't lose weight are just fooling themselves. Maybe they have cut out breakfast. Maybe they make do with a tiny helping of cottage cheese or tuna salad for lunch. And maybe they even manage to deprive themselves of seconds at the dinner table. But if they're not losing weight, they're eating too much.

If that's you, then try keeping a food diary. That means writing down *everything* you eat throughout the day—not just at mealtime. Every cookie you sneak from someone's desk, every glass of soda (unless it's diet soda), every little snack you grab after work or before bed—everything that goes in your mouth has to be recorded. After a few days of doing this—honestly—you may begin to see where those calories are coming from.

Next step is to analyze *why* you're eating. Do you find that you eat the most when you're upset, or nervous, or excited? Does a fight with your boss or spouse send you to the refrigerator? Do you like to munch on a bag of pretzels while you're watching TV?

The only way to overcome this kind of reflexive eating is to substitute something else. Exercise is a great way to work off an attack of anger or frustration. But there are food addictions that require more than a brisk walk or a three-mile jog. One source of help is an organization called Overeaters Anonymous, which is designed to do for compulsive eaters what Alcoholics Anonymous does for drinkers and Gamblers Anonymous does for casino addicts.

Is OA the answer for everyone? No. Nothing is right for everyone. But if it sounds worth trying, you can get in touch with them at Overeaters Anonymous, World Service Office, 2190 190th Street, Torrance, CA 90504.

Ideal Weights

The trouble with most weight charts we've seen is that they divide the population into people with small, medium, and large frames, and then they don't tell you how to figure out which you are. So if your weight looks too high on the medium frame column, say, you can just say to yourself, "I guess I have a large frame." And behold—you're not overweight after all!

Here's a simple test to tell you which frame you have: Measure the circumference of your wrist. For women, 5½ inches or less means a small frame, between 5½ and 6¼ inches is medium, and over 6¼ inches is large. Men should add 1¼ inches to those figures.

This table gives desirable weight ranges for adults, in indoor clothing weighing five pounds including shoes with 1″ heels.

Height	Small frame	Medium frame	Large frame
MEN			
5′ 2″	128-134	131-141	138-150
3″	130-136	133-143	140-153
4″	132-138	135-145	142-156
5″	134-140	137-148	144-160
6″	136-142	139-151	146-164
7″	138-145	142-154	149-168
8″	140-148	145-157	152-172
9″	142-151	148-160	155-176
10″	144-154	151-163	158-180
11″	146-157	154-166	161-184
6′ 0″	149-160	157-170	164-188
1″	152-164	160-174	168-192

6' 2"	155-168	164-178	172-197
3"	158-172	167-182	176-202
4"	162-176	171-187	181-207

WOMEN

4' 10"	102-111	109-121	118-131
11"	103-113	111-123	120-134
5' 0"	104-115	113-126	122-137
1"	106-118	115-129	125-140
2"	108-121	118-132	128-143
3"	111-124	121-135	131-147
4"	114-127	124-138	134-151
5"	117-130	127-141	137-155
6"	120-133	130-144	140-159
7"	123-136	133-147	143-163
8"	126-139	136-150	146-167
9"	129-142	139-153	149-170
10"	132-145	142-156	152-173
11"	135-148	145-159	155-176
6' 0"	138-151	148-162	158-179

Source: Metropolitan Life Insurance Company

Section III - Substance Abuse

We've chosen to limit this section to the four substances that you, as an executive, are most likely to be tempted to abuse: tobacco, alcohol, marijuana, and cocaine. There are others—prescription drugs, heroin, and LSD and other hallucinogens. But relatively few management level people are still dropping acid, popping uppers, or shooting heroin.

Relatively a whole lot, though, are drinking too much, smoking too much, and experimenting too much with cocaine. Drug addiction can happen to corporate chairmen of the board just as easily as it happens to skid row bums. Nor does being in good health in every other respect protect you. If you run a marathon, and then go puff on a cigarette, you undo a lot of good from the running.

Of the four substances, alcohol is in a slightly different category from the others. The experts (unless they work for a tobacco company) are in agreement about cigarettes, marijuana, and cocaine: They're bad for you, and no amount can be considered safe. But alcohol isn't that cut and dry.

Some scientists say that a little alcohol—one or two drinks a day—can actually be beneficial. One possible way: The booze seems to raise the level of HDL cholesterol in the blood. (For more about HDLs, see Chapter 18.) If this is true, and we still aren't certain that it is, then moderate drinkers might be at less risk of heart disease than total abstainers.

But this shouldn't be taken as an endorsement of drinking. The risks of alcohol are far more convincingly established than are the possible benefits. Some people can't take even one drink without seriously impairing their ability to drive, for example. There isn't any controversy about the wisdom of mixing alcohol and driving. There are just rationalizations, and statistics. Like this one: 25,000 people die every year in the U.S. because they thought they could beat the odds.

Warning: The Surgeon General Is Right

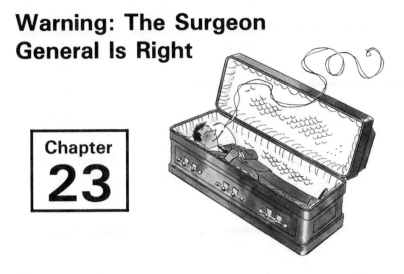

If you smoke cigarettes, you owe it to yourself to know what they can do to you.

Cigarettes are killers. You've heard it before. Every year, thousands upon thousands of Americans die sooner than they would if they hadn't smoked cigarettes. Cigarette smoking has been called the leading preventable cause of premature death among adult Americans. It is responsible to a great extent for the two main causes of early death: heart disease and cancer.

With dire warnings like these in mind, some 30 million Americans have managed to kick the cigarette habit. But another 55 million haven't, though the majority of them say they've tried to quit at least once, and they'd like to quit for good. In the next chapter we'll give some tips on quitting. In this chapter, we want to go over some of the reasons you should.

According to the American Cancer Society, a 25-year-old who smokes two packs a day shortens his or her life by an average of 8.3 years. Here are the ways it happens:

• *Heart attacks.* Cigarettes cause one-quarter of all deaths from heart attack. About 120,000 people die of heart disease each year because they're cigarette smokers.

• *Lung cancer.* Cigarettes cause three-fourths of the cases of lung cancer. Lung cancer is the leading cause of cancer death in this country. Lung cancer is fatal in 90 percent of all cases.

• *Other cancers.* Smoking is *the* cause of 20 percent of all cancer, and *one* of the causes of a third of cancer *deaths*. Smokers are up to 18 times more likely to get cancer of the larynx as nonsmokers, and they face higher risk of cancer of the mouth, esophagus, bladder, and pancreas. If they drink alcohol, the risk increases still more.

• *Respiratory diseases.* Smokers face up to 25 times the risk of dying from bronchitis and emphysema as nonsmokers. Cigarettes cause about 70 percent of the cases of these diseases.

• *Ulcers.* People who smoke cigarettes increase their risk of getting ulcers and their risk of dying from them. Ulcers kill 8,000 Americans each year.

Beyond what cigarettes do to smokers, they pose risks to others as well. Pregnant women who smoke, especially past the fourth month, reduce the amount of oxygen to their babies, and increase the chance of stillbirth, birth defects, and low birth weight. Nonsmokers who must breathe the air around smokers have higher than normal incidence of some of the same diseases smokers get. And cigarette smoking is the leading cause of fatal fires— 2,500 people killed every year.

Even when it doesn't kill, smoking is harmful. It shortens the breath, impairs sleep, causes chronic coughing and spitting, and can hasten the onset of menopause. And smoking causes bad breath (which, to judge by some TV commercials, is a fate *worse* than death!).

But the good news is that the smoking habit, like any other, can be broken. In Chapter 24, we'll show you how to do it.

Quitting Cigarettes: You Can Do It

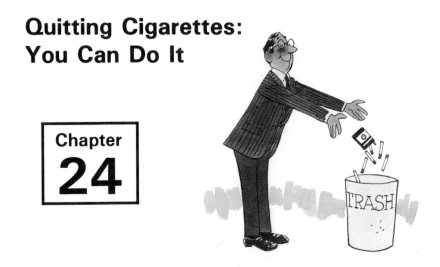

Chapter

24

*If you __really__ want to stop smoking,
you're __already__ halfway there.*

Few subjects arouse people's passions as much as cigarette smoking. People who never smoked or who gave it up are never neutral—they're violently opposed to that filthy weed. People who smoke are just as violently belligerent about defending their habit. Most of them wish they could quit. They just don't think they can.

They're wrong. They can quit—no matter how long they've been smoking, how much they smoke, and how hooked by tobacco they think they are. Anyone who really wants to quit, can. More than 30 million Americans have. But you smoke for yourself, and the only way you can quit is by doing that for yourself. If you try to do it to pacify a spouse or impress your friends, you will almost certainly fail in the long run.

To quit smoking for yourself, you first have to figure out *why* you're about to do this painful, wrenching, agonizing thing to yourself. What do you hope to accomplish by quitting? What kind of positive changes will you expect to achieve by taking cigarette smoke out of your life? Maybe you'd like to become better at some sport or exercise, and you feel that not smoking will help. (It will.) Maybe you enjoy fine dining and you think you'll heighten your sense of taste for food after you get rid of the taste of tobacco. (Right again.) Maybe you're tired of feeling that you're controlled by those little white sticks, and you want to show that you're in charge of your life. (Good for you!) Or maybe you don't want to have to worry about all those diseases that smokers risk getting. So you're taking the plunge.

It's important, as you get ready to quit smoking, that you look on it as a *beginning*—of your life as a nonsmoker —rather than the *end* of your smoking days. What you're doing is adding something positive to your life, not taking something away. You're adding clean air to your lungs, life-giving oxygen to your blood, and probably years to your life.

There are as many formulas for actually stopping smoking as there are former smokers. What worked for your neighbor or your spouse may not work for you. Smoking is an extremely personal pursuit, and the only way to stop it is by finding what is right for you. Here are some tips that can help:

• Do you smoke as a way to get going? To quit, you should find a substitute for cigarettes' stimulation— something like a brisk walk before work, deep breathing, a nourishing bite to eat. Or whatever works for *you.*

• Do you smoke to relieve tension or anxiety? You

probably don't think you could make it through tough situations without your crutch. But you can. Other people, who possess no special abilities you don't have, do it all the time. They use many substitutes—exercise, yoga, an interesting hobby—to name a few. Avoid the temptation to use food as your tension-reliever.

• Are you addicted to smoking? Has smoking lost all pleasurable effects, and do you just continue because you can't do without it? When you're ready to *try* doing without it, quit cold-turkey. For a few days, life will seem unbearable. Hang on. At the end of the torture is a life of freedom from being dominated by a habit you know can do you no good. At the end of a few days of agony are years of satisfaction—the satisfaction that comes from knowing you faced a threat to your health and happiness, and you beat it.

If you want to find out more about breaking the smoking habit, there are several sources of help: The American Cancer Society, the American Lung Association, the American Health Foundation, and Smok-Enders, to name a few. Friends and relatives who have kicked the habit are another good source of inspiration.

But, as we say, it's a very personal thing. You've got to have some good long talks with yourself. Decide you're really ready to quit. Decide how *you* can do it, and why *you* want to. Decide you deserve it. And reward yourself with some extravagant little gift when you succeed.

Nothing can stop you.

An Alcoholic? Me?!

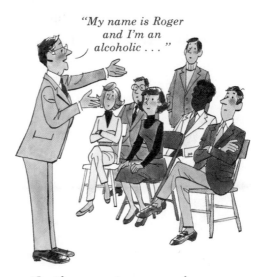

"My name is Roger and I'm an alcoholic . . ."

Alcoholism is a disease that's easy to recognize—in other people. When it comes to ourselves, things aren't so clear.

> *Make not thyself helpless in drinking in the beer shop. For will not the words of thy report repeatedly slip out from thy mouth without thy knowing. Falling down, thy limbs will be broken, and no one will give thee a hand to help thee up. Thy companions will say, "Outside with this drunkard."*
> —Egyptian warning, circa 1500 B.C.

For as long as people have been "drinking in the beer shop", some of them have been drinking too much. But alcoholism is probably the hardest disease in the world for its victims to face up to. Even family and friends, who may welcome the alcoholic's high spirits, are often reluctant to see any connection to alcohol.

Who gets alcoholism? Isn't it a disease of skid-row bums? Respectable business men and women may over-indulge now and then, but they're not the ones who become *alcoholics*, are they?

That's what we used to think. But the truth is that alcoholism is a disease that cuts across all lines of class, age, intelligence, wealth, and occupation. This country has 10 million alcoholics, and only one in 20 is a "skid-row bum".

That doesn't mean that anyone who occasionally goes to a party and gets plastered is an alcoholic. The main thing to watch for is *control*. Who's in charge, you or the booze? If you go someplace intending to have two or three drinks, when you've had that much can you stop? Or do you tend to get drunk almost every time you drink?

What about frequency—is your inebriation becoming more and more common? A social drinker may have too much on rare occasions, but the time to beware is when uncontrolled drinking becomes the rule rather than the exception.

According to one recovered alcoholic, "The drinker is headed for trouble when alcohol becomes a route to ful-fillment, when it's used to produce feelings of superiority, self-confidence, ego strength, happiness, romance, aggressiveness, or any feelings not natural to the drinker's personality."

Abrupt personality changes are a key warning sign: The person who is ordinarily quiet and shy becomes the life of the party. Someone who normally follows the rules and acts responsibly turns into a who-gives-a-damn show-off. The guy who was neat becomes a slob.

But as we said before, alcoholics are experts at denying their disease. And they have a whole list of rationalizations:

"I never drink before dinner." (It's not *when* that counts—it's whether you can control it once you've started.)

"I only drink beer." (You can be an alcoholic just by drinking cough medicine.)

"I'm too young." (There are 12-year-old alcoholics.)

"I can quit any time I want." (That's fine—but *do* you want to quit? If alcohol is what keeps you going, you may not be able to do without it.)

Alcoholism can't be cured. But it can be controlled—all you have to do is stop drinking completely. The hardest part is admitting that your drinking has become a problem. And that you need help to stop.

Help is available from many sources, chief among them Alcoholics Anonymous. AA, an organization that has established an enviable reputation for helping alcoholics recognize and beat their addiction, has chapters throughout the country. In addition, some companies have set up programs for assisting employees who have a drinking problem. Or you can contact local family service agencies, mental health associations, hospital social service departments, or the United Way. And by all means, ask your family physician for advice.

What about a close friend or family member who you think is having a drinking problem—what can you do for them? It's a delicate problem, which we discuss in the next chapter.

Living With an Alcoholic

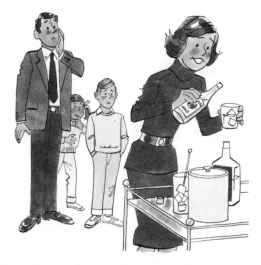

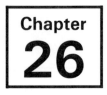

The average alcoholic affects four other people.
That's 50 million people in the U.S.

The alcoholics who are thrown in jail for public drunkenness are not the ones who do the most harm. Ninety percent of them aren't part of a family, so their drinking, for the most part, hurts only themselves.

By contrast, most alcoholics are outwardly normal in most respects, and their drinking usually doesn't land them in jail. These are the "social drinkers" who just like to have an occasional one or two drinks to loosen up. The trouble is, too often the one or two they say they're going to have turn into five or six. They can't control their drinking—any more than the bowery bum can. But their kind of drinking is accepted by society, and it keeps on getting worse. And in the process, these alcoholics are hurting others besides themselves.

—They're hurting their employers. Industry losses related to alcoholism include absenteeism, accidents, and reduced productivity—and most alcoholics are long-service employees who would be expensive to replace.

—They're hurting people on the road. Half of all auto accidents involve alcohol, and half of those involve an alcoholic.

Most important, they're hurting their families. Spouses may find themselves blamed for everything that is wrong in an alcoholic marriage—and they may come to believe it's true. Children lose the love and companionship of an alcoholic parent who is immersed in his or her addiction —and they grow up with a model of adult drunkenness to shape their future behavior.

It is the nature of alcoholism to lock its victims into a pattern of denying that anything is wrong, and resisting offers of help. But the family of the problem drinker needn't stand by helplessly and let their own lives be destroyed. Compassion means showing the willingness to suffer *with* someone—but it doesn't mean suffering alone because of that person's unwillingness to suffer. First, learn all you can about the disease—from Alcoholics Anonymous, the National Council on Alcoholism, or local hospitals and mental health centers. Al-Anon and Alateen, groups devoted specifically to helping the families of alcoholics, provide practical guidance on living with an alcoholic.

Here are some general guidelines:

1. Don't preach, nag, lecture, or assume a holier-than-thou attitude; this will only cause the alcoholic to retreat further into the bottle. Instead, show plenty of love and

encouragement for every small improvement.

2. Don't cover up. Let the alcoholic experience the consequences of his actions, even when those consequences seem cruel and humiliating. The only way to get someone to kick a bad habit is by letting the bad part come through.

3. Don't hide bottles or pour liquor down the sink. You'll just force the alcoholic to establish a secret supply. Liquor is available everywhere; if someone wants a drink, he will find it. An alcoholic won't stop drinking until he himself decides he must.

4. Don't argue with the drinker when he's drunk. The response may be evasion, deceit, or even anger and violence. Approach him when he's sober, or during a hangover, when the unpleasant effects of alcohol are most apparent.

5. Don't make vague threats; instead, set specific limits on the person's drinking. Insist that those limits be adhered to every time, and if there is to be some consequence of exceeding the limits, make sure you follow through.

6. Don't expect instant results. Al-Anon and Alateen can provide vital support and guidance. But alcoholism is a serious disease, and some people just aren't capable of overcoming it. It is essential that you, the spouse or child or parent or friend, not blame yourself for the person's addiction. The worst tragedy is when those who love the victim of this disease allow their love to drag them down with the alcoholic.

Marijuana—Is It Really the Safe Drug?

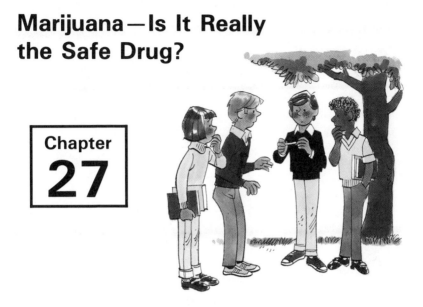

Chapter
27

Is grass really a harmless little weed,
like the kids keep saying?

It took a half century of heavy cigarette smoking by millions of Americans before the serious hazards posed by tobacco were recognized, so it's not too surprising that we know relatively little about marijuana at this point. In spite of the fact that one out of three adult Americans have tried grass, and two-thirds of all young adults use it at least occasionally, the drug is relatively new to the scene. But, while there are still some doubts about some of its risks, we do know more now than we did back in the 60's, when the flower children were beckoning everyone to "tune in, turn on, and drop out".

If you know 20 teenagers, the odds are that five or six of them smoke marijuana regularly. One out of nine high school seniors uses pot every day. Investigators say the drug is even showing up increasingly in grammar schools all over the country. And if there's one thing about which we're certain concerning marijuana, it is that the younger the user, the higher the risk.

Those risks can be broken down into two groups: the effects on a person during a "high", and the long-term hazards to habitual users.

Immediate Effects

Someone high on grass behaves in many ways like someone drunk on alcohol. In particular, marijuana impairs perception of time and space, memory, learning ability, speech, reading comprehension, and the ability to think. It goes without saying that driving ability is dangerously affected, along with general intellectual performance. Reaction time is slower, coordination is decreased, and people who can normally operate complicated machinery may be unable to do so while high on grass. The problem is that those people may *think* they can still function normally. Finally, there's always a risk of a panic reaction to a high—a "bad trip". Hospital emergency rooms are getting used to treating people suffering from adverse marijuana reactions.

Long Term Effects

While the immediate effects of grass are readily apparent and well documented, the long term effects are still uncertain. But recent research has pointed to the likelihood of a significant risk in several areas:

• *Lung damage.* Most marijuana users smoke considerably less than those who smoke tobacco, but they still face the same kind of risks. One study showed that five marijuana cigarettes smoked over a week would cause more lung damage than six packs of tobacco cigarettes. Among the forms that damage takes are irritation of the air passages, reduction of lung capacity, impaired defense against infection, and extensive lung inflammation. Regular users increase their risk of bronchitis and emphysema. It is too early to say whether smoking marijuana leads to lung cancer. But the smoke of grass contains 150 chemicals, most of whose effects are unknown. Common sense indicates that at least some of them will turn out to cause cancer.

• *Heart effects.* Young, healthy people probably don't face any life-threatening heart damage from marijuana. But those who already have heart problems may suffer increased angina—the chest pain that often signals a heart attack.

• *Reproductive effects.* Several studies have shown that marijuana may have an adverse effect on male and female fertility. And when pregnant women smoke, the marijuana can get into the unborn fetus's blood supply. The full implications of this are not yet known, but it is known that marijuana users have more miscarriages than nonusers.

• *Other.* There is some evidence to suggest that marijuana damages the body's defense against disease— the immune system. An adverse effect on the hypothalamus—the body's master gland—is also suspected.

If anyone needs any more reasons to avoid pot smoking, there's one more fact, and this one's indisputable: Marijuana is still illegal.

Cocaine: The Flight to Nowhere

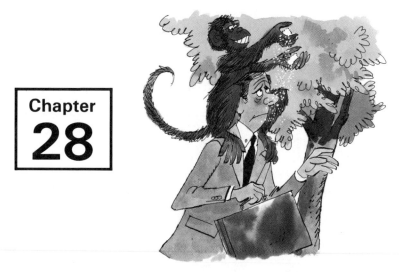

Chapter
28

Cocaine—it may be "in", but don't let it get in you.

To speak of cocaine abuse in the United States as an epidemic is to tell only part of the story. People who have no exposure to the drug can't really comprehend the extent to which coke has infested everyday life. But consider:

• The traffic in cocaine is put at some 45 tons a year. The price tag for this mountain of snow: $25 billion.

• Five million Americans use coke regularly, and a quarter of them are dependent on the drug.

• Cocaine is not limited to trendy suburbanites, professional athletes, or high-living show-biz types. The drug is used by people in *all* walks of life.

That's the scary part. People you'd never suspect of having a drug habit are spending huge chunks of their salaries—and whatever other money they can get their hands on—for cocaine. Police officers. Doctors. Airline pilots. Lawyers. White-collar workers in every kind of business, who appear "normal" but who have the monkey of a cocaine dependency on their backs.

What is the allure of cocaine? It varies with the user, and can range from the need for a physical pick-me-up on Monday mornings at work to a desire to keep up with the latest trend. Lots of coke users start out by inhaling a few "lines" of the white powder at a party. Typically, they enjoy the experience, find that they're still able to function normally the next day, and start looking for the next opportunity. For many, snorting the powder eventually gives way to a more potent method of getting high —free-basing, which is smoking a concentrated mixture of cocaine and ether in a water pipe.

While an addiction to cocaine can lead to serious physical problems, such as liver and lung damage, severe weight loss, and even heart attacks, the main risk isn't medical. It's financial. If you use those figures above—5 million cokeheads spending $25 billion a year—you come up with $5,000 per user. That's high enough, but it's just an average. Some people spend a thousand dollars *a week*. People who develop serious addiction to coke frequently cash their paychecks and head for the local dealer to buy as much cocaine as they can get. Whatever's left will go to pay the mortgage and other bills.

When the weekly paycheck isn't enough, many coke users turn to theft. If they're kids, they may steal money from their parents. If they're adults in a position to get money from their employers, they often resort to some form of embezzlement. If they have no other alternative, they may just turn to common burglary or robbery. Or murder, if that becomes necessary.

Drug experts and law-enforcement officials are in basic agreement about one point: Cocaine use is not being controlled by scare tactics or by legal crackdowns. The attraction is too great. For the sales rep who has to be "up" for every customer presentation, a snort of coke looks like the perfect answer. For the truck driver under pressure to get his rig across the country in a hurry, cocaine keeps him at the wheel. For the advertising copywriter, a hit of high-quality free-base seems to fire up the creative juices and gets the job done.

Many of these people can continue normal lives, even while using more and more cocaine. Many of them outgrow their desire for the drug, and stop on their own.

But others are not so lucky. For a growing number of coke users, a little now and then becomes a lot, all the time. A habit that started out costing $25 or $50 a week eventually claims thousands of dollars. The need to get that kind of money becomes the force that directs everything the addict does. The process is complete—cocaine has taken over completely.

Section IV - Major Diseases

This is a health book, not a disease book. We're interested in showing you how to make the lifestyle changes that will improve your overall health and fitness, not in showing you how to cure yourself when you get sick.

Still, preventing and treating diseases is part of the story. When you start an exercise program, it is to be hoped that you're acting at least partly out of a desire to feel good and have fun. But there's also an element of "this is a good way to cut my chances of a heart attack" in there.

This section will give you some of the basics about five of the diseases most likely to have a major impact on your life. We'll go into prevention, treatment, and, where there *is* one, cure. We'll try to help you live with chronic diseases like heart diease and diabetes.

And, in our chapter on the holiday blues, we'll try to give you some ideas to avoid depression. It's a disease, believe it or not. A lot of medical research has been done on depression, and doctors are becoming convinced that depression is more than a state of mind—it can be the result of a chemical imbalance that is often treatable by drugs. It's also treatable by exercise. Amazing what a little sweat can do, isn't it?

How to Give Your Heart a Fighting Chance

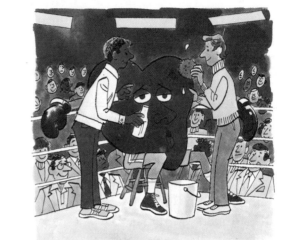

Chapter

29

Want to worry less about a heart attack?
Here's what you have to do.

Why do six hundred thousand Americans die of heart attacks every year? Is it just that "you have to die of something"? A lot of people believe that—they think that if your time has come, you're going to die, and that there's not much you can do to put that day off.

Of course, that's not true. There is plenty you can do to reduce your chance of having a heart attack, and increase your chances of survival if you do have one. Much of what we discuss in the rest of this book is geared toward improving the health of your heart. In this chapter, we'll put it all in one place.

We should point out that the suggestions we make will

not confer total immunity to heart attack. Nothing has yet been found that will do that. Some people face a higher-than-average risk of heart disease no matter how clean a life they live—because of a family history of heart problems. But even they can keep that risk to a minimum if they control the things that are controllable.

Freedom from heart disease is the "payoff" from a series of "bets" you make by the way you live. The more bets you make, the better your chances of winning the payoff. It's never a 100 percent sure thing, but the name of the game is to improve your odds. Here's how:

1. *Control your weight.* Find out what your ideal weight is, and keep within five pounds of that. People who are significantly overweight run the risk of adding extra fat deposits to their arteries, which is one of the causes of heart attacks.

2. *Control blood pressure.* You may have heard of the rule of thumb for determining normal blood pressure— the first number should be 100 plus your age. Well, that's a handy rule, but it's wrong. There's no reason your blood pressure has to get higher as you get older. It *does* for many Americans, because of their unhealthy lifestyles. Aim for 120/80. If it climbs much beyond that, consult your doctor about the best ways to bring it down. If you have been told to take medicine to lower your blood pressure, take it regularly, even when you feel fine. If the medicine produces unwelcome side effects, ask your doctor to prescribe something else. High blood pressure is a major factor in causing heart attacks.

3. *Eat fiber, not fat.* Diets high in saturated fat and cholesterol are likely to clog up your arteries. Eat less of

these: red meats, fried foods, pastries, dairy products (except skim milk), egg yolks. Instead, eat more fresh and frozen fruits and vegetables, whole-grain cereals and bread, and rice and pasta. The fiber in these foods helps lower blood cholesterol and clean out your arteries.

4. *Get regular, aerobic exercise.* When you work up a sweat, you strengthen your heart. You also decrease the harmful cholesterol buildup in your blood and help control your weight. The best exercises are ones you can do at least three times a week, for at least 20 minutes at a time, and that get your pulse up in the 120-140 range for the whole time you're exercising.

5. *No smoking.* Cigarette smoking is thought to be the leading cause of heart attacks. It's also a leading cause of cancer. All in all, an excellent habit to do without.

6. *Reduce blood sugar.* If you're a diabetic, or the doctor says you have high blood sugar, you have to be especially careful to watch your weight and get enough exercise. And you should avoid foods high in all sugars.

7. *Learn how to unwind.* Stress is believed to play a role in heart attack—both directly, by adding to the heart's burden, and indirectly, by elevating blood pressure. If you live a stressful life, you need to find ways to relax. Try exercise, meditation, self-hypnosis, yoga, or dancing.

Following these guidelines will not sentence you to a dreary life of constant self-denial. Give it a try—one step at a time, if that's easier. You may actually find you enjoy living more!

After a Heart Attack— Life Goes On

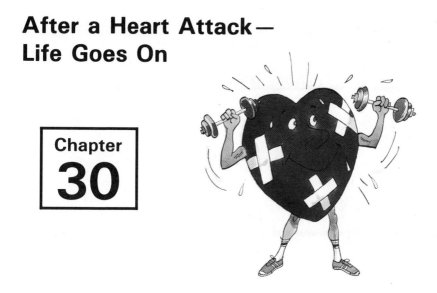

Chapter
30

Sometimes a heart attack can be the start of the best years of a person's life.

One of the brightest success stories in medical science is the survival of people with heart disease. After years of steadily increasing death rates from heart attacks, the trend has reversed. A lot of the credit goes to improved care in the hospital and better drugs. But another reason is a revolution in the way doctors tell people who have survived a heart attack to live their lives.

In the past, heart patients were told to avoid physical exertion, emotional stress, and sexual activity. They were advised that if they wanted to avoid another heart attack they'd have to become, in effect, perpetually inactive. In some cases, they were warned to quit their jobs, since their doctors considered the physical or emotional demands more than they could handle.

We now know that this kind of therapy is appropriate in only the most serious cases. For most patients, the life of an invalid is actually just the kind of thing that *increases* the chance of another attack. The way for a person to prevent a second heart attack, doctors have found, is to do what he or she should have done to prevent the first.

Physical activity: Exercise is one of the best ways to counter the depression that often accompanies heart attacks. The time to begin changing exercise habits is probably before even leaving the hospital—under medical supervision, of course. A heart attack patient who has not exercised before the attack should take things slowly. The doctor can draw up a schedule of gradually increasing activity, or recommend a formal rehabilitation program. The important thing, though, is to build up the muscle that created the problem in the first place—the heart. And the way to do that is by carefully controlled and monitored exercise.

Excitement: If you tell a heart patient to avoid getting excited or worried, the most likely result will be that he'll start worrying about getting worried. At best, he'll deprive himself of the things that make life enjoyable— and for no good reason. Everyone should avoid too much stress, but there's just no sound scientific basis for a person recovering from a heart attack to be concerned about the normal peaks and valleys of daily life.

Sex: There are so many myths about the effects of sexual activity on a person with heart problems that it's no wonder many heart patients become depressed and withdrawn. The truth is this: Sex is no different from other mild forms of physical exertion, and there's no reason normal sexual activity can't continue.

Diet: A lot of heart attacks are the result, at least partially, of eating a lot of the foods you should eat only a little of—such as anything high in fat, especially saturated fat, and fried, greasy foods. Doctors haven't really changed their advice in this area too much—change to a diet of limited fats and plenty of fruits, vegetables, and whole grains. If you're overweight, bring it down gradually.

Smoking: There's only one thing to say to a heart patient who's a cigarette smoker: Stop.

Whatever heart patients do after the attack should be done only in close consultation with their doctor. With the right approach to therapy, there's no limit to what patients can do with the rest of their lives. Literally thousands of men and women who have had heart attacks have turned their lives around. Some even run in marathons!

It sure beats life in a rocking chair.

Is It the Big "C"?

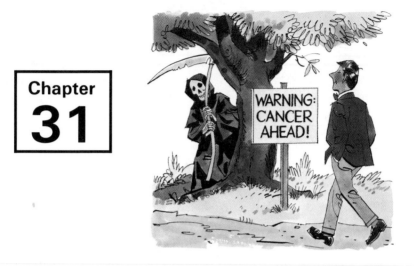

Most cancers give plenty of warning—if we know what to look for.

Cancer, as you may have heard, is not one disease but actually more than 100. Some cancers are more dangerous than others, but all are characterized by uncontrolled growth of the cells from part of the body. People look forward to the day when scientists will find a cure for cancer, but it's unlikely that a single cure will apply to so many different kinds of the disease.

Many doctors are convinced that the best hope for reducing the toll that cancer takes on human lives lies in prevention and early detection. A study by the American Cancer Society has identified some preventive measures everyone can take to minimize the risk of cancer; we'll describe those measures in Chapter 32.

Even the deadliest forms of cancer are often curable, and the rate of cure goes up dramatically when the cancer is discovered early. Sometimes that discovery occurs during a physical examination by a doctor. But how many of us get regular physicals? There's no one in a better position to detect the warning signs of cancer than you.

The major warning signs:

1. *Change in bowel or bladder habits.* If you have trouble going to the bathroom, it could be a sign of cancer of the colon, bladder, or, in men, the prostate gland. Constipation, of course, usually doesn't mean cancer. But if it persists or gets worse, you should see a doctor and have the problem checked out.

2. *A persistent sore, wart, or mole.* If you notice a raised, irregular area like a wart in your cheek, gum, or tongue, it could be a sign of cancer of the mouth—one of the most easily treatable forms of cancer, if diagnosed in time. Skin cancer can appear as a sore that doesn't heal in a reasonable amount of time; a dry, scaly patch or pimple that doesn't go away; or a dark brown or black mole-like growth that becomes larger, bleeds, or changes color. Show it to your doctor.

3. *Unusual bleeding or discharge.* Any abnormal bleeding or discharge of fluids from the vagina can be a sign of cancer of the uterus. (The best way to find early uterine cancer is still the Pap test, a simple procedure that doctors administer.) Blood in the stool may mean cancer of the colon or rectum—or just bleeding hemorrhoids. Get it checked out anyway to be safe.

4. *Thickening or lump in the breast or elsewhere.*

Every woman should know how to examine her breasts once a month to detect lumps as early as possible. Most such lumps are *not* cancer, and even the ones that are malignant need not mean death or disfiguring surgery. Many doctors now treat breast cancer without removing the whole breast, and, as with other cancers, the earlier it's found, the better the success rate.

5. *Indigestion or difficulty in swallowing.* This may consist of a sense of general discomfort or mild pain in the stomach, fullness or bloating, slight nausea, heartburn, loss of appetite, burping, or vomiting. Obviously, these symptoms usually don't signal cancer. It's when they persist or get worse that you should have them checked out.

6. *Nagging cough or hoarseness.* A persistent cough could mean lung cancer. Coughs that seem to hang on should be checked out, especially if you're a cigarette smoker. Hoarseness, a lump in the throat, or soreness in the neck can be warnings of cancer of the larynx (the vocal cords). With early diagnosis and treatment the rate of cure is high.

7. *Unexplained weight loss.* Many people are so grateful for any weight loss that they ignore this signal. But it could mean cancer of the stomach, pancreas, or intestine.

How important is it to know these warning signs and to act on them? Consider this: More than 100,000 people who die of cancer every year would have lived if they had caught the disease in time. No one wants to hear the doctor say, "It's cancer." But if you heed the body's early warning system, the doctor's report is more likely to be, "It's cancer, and we can cure it."

Cancer: What We Know About Prevention

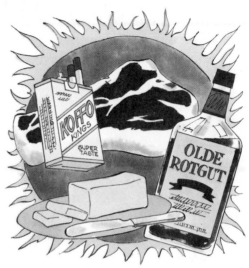

It's easier to prevent cancer than to cure it.

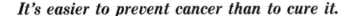

Hardly a week goes by, it seems, without yet another warning from the government that some chemical pesticide or food additive has been found to cause cancer. Small wonder that many people have concluded that *everything* causes cancer, and that there's not a thing they can do about it.

Of course, the truth is that everything *doesn't* cause cancer. Most things don't. The chemicals and pollutants that have stirred up the most publicity cause only a small fraction of all cancers in the U.S. And, contrary to what the fatalists have concluded, there is plenty that individuals can do to reduce their risk.

In spite of the dread associated with cancer, surprisingly few people have any idea of what they can do to minimize their chances of getting it. According to the National Cancer Institute, only about one person in six has ever been given cancer-prevention advice by a physician, though a majority of those surveyed said they'd follow such advice.

The recommendations outlined here represent the best that medical science can come up with at this time. Naturally, even following every suggestion to the letter won't give you 100 percent immunity from all forms of cancer. But the NCI estimates that 100,000 people each year could be saved if Americans adopted these lifestyle changes.

1. *No smoking.* Smoking greatly increases your risk of cancer of the lung, larynx, esophagus, pancreas, bladder, kidney, cervix, and mouth. As soon as you quit your body begins to repair the damage, and in time you can be as risk-free as someone who never smoked.

2. *Go easy on alcohol.* One or two drinks a day should be your limit. More than that increases your risk of cancer of the mouth, throat, esophagus, and liver.

3. *Control your weight.* Anything more than a few pounds overweight increases your risk of cancer of the colon.

4. *Less fat.* Cutting back on fatty red meats and dairy products lowers your risk of breast and colon cancer. Instead of these, try to eat . . .

5. . . . *more fiber.* The best sources are most fruits, vegetables, and whole-grain cereals. Especially bene-

ficial are dark green vegetables and citrus fruits. Some studies have singled out a significant anti-cancer effect from eating cabbage, broccoli, and brussels sprouts.

6. *Avoid unneeded X-rays.* Don't ask for X-rays your doctor hasn't recommended. Make sure you wear a lead apron when the dentist X-rays your mouth.

7. *Caution on the job.* If your job occasionally puts you in contact with carcinogenic substances, use the protective devices and clothing your company provides.

8. *Block the sun.* Too much exposure to the sun, especially at midday in the summer, is a major cause of skin cancer. If you can't stay in the shade, use a sunscreen with a Skin Protection Factor of 10-15.

9. *Estrogen: lower the dose.* Women who take estrogen supplements for relief of menopausal symptoms should take the medication only as long as necessary. Lowering the dose of estrogen, and combining it with progesterone, reduces the risk of cancer of the uterus, ovaries, and breast.

How important are these preventive steps? Just look at a few statistics. Every year, cancer strikes 870,000 Americans. Of those, more than 600,000 are caused by one or more of these factors that individuals can control.

We don't know how to cure all cancer yet.

But we do know how to prevent most cancer. It's in your power.

What's Your B.P.?

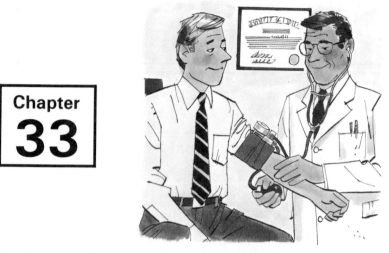

Chapter
33

The first step in controlling high blood pressure is knowing you have it.

Everyone knows that high blood pressure—doctors call it hypertension—is bad. But what is high blood pressure? How do you get it? How can you prevent it? If you get it, is it curable? And what can high blood pressure do to you? Not only don't most people know the answers to those questions, most people have no idea what their own blood pressure is.

High blood pressure is widespread—about one of three adult Americans has it. The biggest problem, though, is that most of them don't know it. Hypertension has no symptoms. The first sign of high blood pressure is often the onset of one of the diseases it can help cause, including heart disease, stroke, and kidney failure.

High blood pressure is what you have when your heart has to push too hard to move your blood. Think of a water pump that has to pump a steady stream of water up a hill, through a thin hose with lots of kinks.

Your heart wants to keep a steady stream of blood circulating throughout your body, but sometimes things go wrong and the job becomes harder. When something upsets the normal balance of fluids—one of the consequences of too much salt—the supply of blood can build up too high. That boosts the pressure. Or the problem can lie with your blood vessels—the arteries and veins that transport the blood from the heart to every part of the body. If those vessels get clogged by deposits of fat or plaque, the heart has to work harder to push the same amount of blood through narrower tubes.

Some people think that the term "hypertension" means that high blood pressure only happens to people who are tense. Not so. The disease can strike people who are calm, stress-free, and without any outward sign of trouble. It strikes people of all ages, though older people are more at risk. It strikes men and women, but men suffer more fatalities from hypertension than women. Whites and blacks both get high blood pressure, but blacks get it more often.

Besides age, sex, and race, there are other factors that increase your risk of high blood pressure: being overweight, a diet that's too high in salt, smoking, not enough exercise, and the wrong parents. (If your parents had high blood pressure, your risk is higher.)

You can't do anything about your heredity, but you can reduce your chances of developing hypertension by making the appropriate changes in your lifestyle—keep your weight at the proper level, cut down on salt, stay away from cigarettes, and get regular aerobic exercise.

And there's another step you can take that won't keep you from getting hypertension, but it could save your life—get your blood pressure checked. The fact is, almost all high blood pressure is treatable. But only if it's discovered.

If you're diagnosed as having high blood pressure, the first thing to keep in mind is that you haven't been handed a death sentence. Hypertension is readily treatable by several methods. The first is those lifestyle changes. Another is drug therapy—drugs for the treatment of high blood pressure are highly effective, as long as the patient keeps taking them. Sometimes the drugs will produce unpleasant side effects, and patients may stop taking them without consulting the doctor. That's a mistake. There are several effective medicines available, and a change in prescription may be all that's needed to prevent the side effects.

A third form of treatment is to do what you can to limit the risk of the diseases that high blood pressure helps cause. For example, you might cut down on high-fat and high-cholesterol foods to reduce your risk of heart disease. And you might do your kidneys a favor by limiting your alcohol consumption.

But the first step is to find out what your blood pressure is. Normal for adults is about 120 over 80, which represents the pressure during the heart's contraction and the pressure when the heart is relaxed. Children's readings should be about 15 percent lower. It only takes your doctor a minute or so to check your blood pressure. You can even do it yourself by buying your own sphygmomanometer. Hard to pronounce, but easy to use. And maybe a lifesaver.

Diabetes: Living Without Sugar

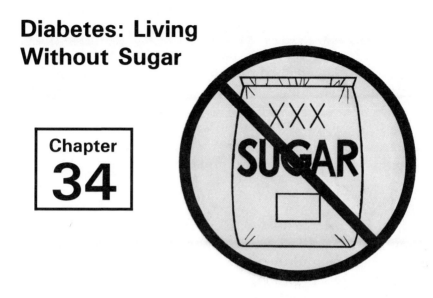

Chapter
34

It's not curable—yet. But you can learn to live with it.

There was a time when all diabetics faced an early death. Then artificial insulin was developed to control the disease, and a lot of diabetics got a new lease on life.

But diabetes is still a serious disease. It's the third highest cause of death by disease (after heart disease and cancer) in the U.S. It's a major contributor to such other health problems as blindness, heart disease, and atherosclerosis—hardening of the arteries. And people with the most serious forms of diabetes have lifespans as much as a third shorter than the general population.

Most people know that diabetics have to restrict their sugar intake, but beyond that there's a lot of misunderstanding. Here are some basics:

Q.: What is diabetes?

A.: It's a group of chronic diseases affecting the way

the body uses energy. Type I diabetes is the more serious, and begins in childhood or early adulthood. The symptoms include frequent urination accompanied by abnormal thirst, sudden weight loss, and frequent cravings for sweets. Type II generally appears in middle age or later. The signs of this form of the disease may include those for Type I, as well as frequent drowsiness, blurred vision, and tingling or numbness in the feet.

Q.: What is the role of insulin?

A.: Insulin, a hormone produced by the pancreas, enables the cells to use sugars in the blood for energy. In diabetics, something goes wrong with that system—either there's not enough insulin, or there's a disruption in the way the cells use the insulin. In either case, the direct result is too much sugar in the blood.

Q.: What causes diabetes?

A.: Several factors are involved, most of them beyond our control. There's a strong genetic connection—if someone in your family had diabetes, your chances of getting the disease are increased. The disease also strikes women more often than men, and is more prevalent in people over 40. There is one risk factor you can control, though: overweight. Your chances of developing diabetes *double* with every 20 percent of excess weight.

Q.: How is it treated?

A.: An estimated 1.5 million diabetics, mostly those with Type I, have to take daily shots of insulin to control the disease. But millions of others can live with diabetes without the needle. A diet low in fat and high in fiber and complex carbohydrates (fruits, vegetables, and whole-grained cereals) may be the only measure needed. Often the doctor will also recommend an increase in exercise, which helps both by controlling weight and by increasing the body's sensitivity to insulin. For all diabetics, of course, it's essential to cut way down on everything that contains a lot of sugar.

Q.: Is there a cure for diabetes?

A.: No—not yet. But few medical mysteries have been the subject of as much research as diabetes, and the prospect of an eventual cure is very real. Until that day, it is helpful to keep things in perspective. Sure, diabetes is serious. But millions of people live their lives with little or no disruption in spite of the illness. And as it happens, the advice on diet and exercise that's given to diabetics is good advice for everyone.

The Holiday Blues

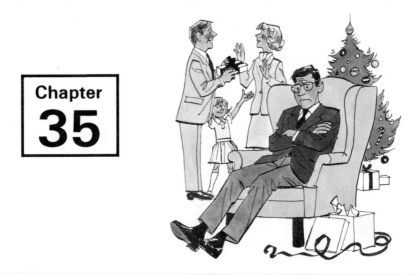

'Tis not necessarily the season to be jolly.

It's a persistent misconception that the holiday season —Thanksgiving, Christmas, Hanukkah, and New Year's—is an automatic spirit booster for everyone. It isn't fair, of course. Advertisers and TV news features gear up for the "happiest time of the year". Parties, gift-giving, cards, family get-togethers—it just isn't fair.

What if you don't have that holiday mood . . . does that make you some kind of antisocial grouch? Is there something seriously wrong with a person who refuses to allow the merriment that everyone else seems to feel to rub off?

There are some very real reasons why lots of people feel down in the dumps amid all the festivities:

- The holidays are supposed to be a time of joy for

everyone. The country reverberates with calls to have fun! Be happy! Be thankful! But people who are having problems in their marriages or family relationships and people who live by themselves may not see any reason to feel joyful. During most of the year these people can ignore their loneliness and depression, but it's hard when so much attention is being paid to families and togetherness.

• The holidays are a time to remember. But some people would just as soon forget. As kids they may have had unhappy Christmases, and the sights, sounds, and smells of the season bring back the misery.

• Some people set themselves up for disappointment by overdoing the gift-giving and party-going. They hope they'll be paid back in love and appreciation, but the results frequently fail to measure up to their expectations.

Depression is one of the most baffling and complicated afflictions we have to deal with. But that doesn't mean it *can't* be dealt with. The first thing to do is realize that, if you feel rotten, you're not alone. Sometimes that realization makes the blues a little easier to bear. Other suggestions:

• *See your doctor.* Depression, whatever time of the year it happens, is a medical problem that can often be treated by drugs, psychotherapy, or other means. If you're taking medicine for heart disease or high blood pressure, it's possible that the drugs are at least partly responsible for your depression. See if your doctor can prescribe something that doesn't produce the side effects.

• *Run away from the problem.* Running, or any other strenuous exercise, is an excellent way to alleviate the

131

blues. Beyond the fact that your mind is off your problems while you're working out, there's actually a chemical basis to this advice. Exercise seems to stimulate the endorphins—chemicals in the brain that act as natural tranquilizers.

• *Lean on friends.* If you live alone or are trapped in an unhappy marriage, friends can give you the human contact you're lacking. The best friends are the people you can share bad times with as well as happy times.

• *Check your menu.* Believe it or not, the food you eat can have an impact on your state of mind. A diet short on B vitamins can deprive the brain of those same mood-elevating chemicals that exercise stimulates. Sources of the B-complex: whole grains, green vegetables, eggs, and fish. Or vitamin pills if you want to supplement your diet.

• *Be good to yourself.* If it seems that the world is passing you by, maybe you should just take care of Number One yourself. This is the time to let budgets and calorie regimens take a back seat to bursts of self-indulgence. If you have the time and money, why not take a vacation in the sun? There are few better ways to brighten a gloomy winter mood than spreading out on some Caribbean beach. Even a weekend trip can work wonders.

Of course, it doesn't have to be something that expensive. How about a bouquet of flowers, from *you* to *you*?

Section V - Stress

If there's one condition that has come to be regarded as an occupational hazard for executives, it's stress. When your job calls for decisions that affect large sums of money and/or large numbers of people, you can't help worrying a little. The trick is not to stop worrying, the trick is to know what to do about it.

The only way to completely eliminate stress is to die, so most of us will have to be content with getting stress under control. In this section we'll give you some pointers. Our chapter on Type A personality will hold up a mirror for you. If you see yourself in the description of Type A, you have a special need to make some changes.

Sometimes stress can cause you to lose sleep. When that happens, you're even less able to deal with the work-related problems that cause your stress than before, so Chapter 38 will try to help you sleep better. If you'd like to try a new approach to stress control, read about self-hypnosis and laughter in Chapters 37 and 39.

Take it easy.

Are You a "Type A"?

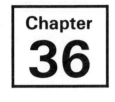

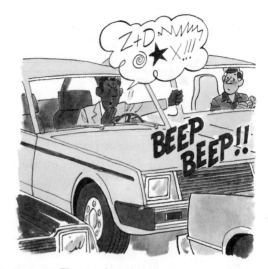

It's not much fun being a Type A person—
or being around one.

It's fine to be hard-working, competitive, and energetic, but some people go too far. You know the type—they're the first to hit their car horn if you don't move fast enough when the light turns green. They get upset if they have to wait for anyone or anything, especially if they don't have something to do while they're waiting. They lose their tempers at minor irritations, like noisy kids or a TV that goes on the blink.

Psychologists say this kind of person has a "Type A" personality. (A Type B person, naturally, is just the opposite—laid back, unhurried, unruffled in even the worst crisis.) And there is convincing evidence to suggest that all this stress is bad for you. The main reasons: It can lead to temporary surges in blood pressure, insomnia, muscle soreness, and heart problems. It can give you an ulcer, frequent headaches, and it often causes people to turn to drugs and alcohol as a way of calming down.

You may feel that stress is a necessary part of your job. You don't especially like it, but that's what you're being paid for. There are degrees of Type A-ness, and it's not so bad to have a certain amount of get-up-and-go. You probably wouldn't want to change completely to a Type B person anyway—even if you could. But there are some relatively easy ways to ease back a bit on the throttle of Type A living.

• Think about what really matters to you. Are the seconds or minutes you save by hurrying through everything that important? Are you devoting your energy to the things that count the most—or spreading yourself too thin on activities that deserve less attention? Do you know when to say yes, and when to delegate?

• Build time into your schedule so you won't have to rush. Get up a littler earlier in the morning to make getting to work less frenzied. Start working on projects *before* the last minute. Finish things before they're due— and enjoy the great feeling it gives you!

• Do you take a coffee break? For a change of pace, why not make it a "relaxation break". Forget the coffee and go somewhere where you won't be disturbed. Put your feet up, and do nothing. Think about some pleasant experience or place, and allow yourself to feel like you're back there again.

• Next time you have nothing particular planned for lunch, why not leave it that way! Make it a light meal, followed by whatever you feel like doing. Go for a walk. Lie down somewhere and think about your special place or experience. Talk to some people you don't normally spend time with. Read a good book. Anything *you* feel like doing.

• Any time you think you might have to wait—in line, for an appointment, in a traffic jam—bring along something to make the delay more pleasant, like a book, a favorite music tape, some unfinished letters or unpaid bills. Or, if you can, bring along a *person* you like.

• Force yourself to slow down. If you find you're passing everyone on the road, even when you're not in that big a hurry, bring it back down to the speed limit and move over to the right-hand lane. Let the others pass you for a change. You'll be surprised to find that you live through the experience!

• Don't get upset about things you can't do anything about. No matter how mad you get at the bus or train that's late, it won't come any earlier. It's OK to tell yourself you'll never come back to the store whose salesclerks don't know what they're doing, but getting mad about it doesn't help at all. Save your anger for important matters—and things you can change.

• After work, when you have some free time, spend some of it by yourself, doing nothing. Find a nice quiet place where you can't be disturbed, take your watch off so you can't keep track of time, and just sit back and daydream. If you're not used to this, it can take a little getting used to. Your first reaction may be to feel guilty about wasting time. But the time you spend with no one but yourself, doing nothing at all, can sometimes be the most pleasant, refreshing part of your day.

How to Hypnotize Yourself

Chapter

37

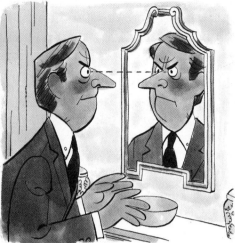

There's no trick to learning self-hypnosis.

When most people think of hypnosis, they picture a strong-willed, Svengali-type person imposing his or her will on someone else. Remember the comic strip "Mandrake the Magician"? All Mandrake had to do to take control of his powerless victims' minds was stare into their eyes and "gesture hypnotically".

Or you may have watched a night club hypnotist who professed to be able to put members of the audience in a trance so deep they would do whatever he commanded— bark like a dog, for example. But more and more, hypnosis is changing its image and becoming a respectable therapeutic procedure, a way to help people who want to make changes in their behavior.

A lot of people have used hypnosis to help quit smoking

or lose weight. But it can do a lot more. Some experts feel that hypnosis can help people do almost anything they want to do, from overcoming a fear of public speaking to playing better tennis. And it's an excellent way to reduce tension.

That point is worth repeating: Hypnosis helps you do what you *want* to do. Hypnosis will *not* change your personality, nor can it make you do something harmful to yourself or others, nor can it make you lose control of your mind. Hypnosis, in fact, is a way for you to *gain* control of your mind.

Hypnosis is nothing more than a form of relaxation that enables you to communicate with your subconscious mind. Since the subconscious mind affects almost everything you do, it follows that hypnosis can have broad applications.

If you're interested in learning hypnosis, you may be able to find an adult education course on the subject. Or you can ask friends or your doctor to recommend a reliable professional hypnotherapist. Or you can start with this simple procedure.

STEP ONE: Find a quiet place. You should use self-hypnosis only at times and in places you can be completely relaxed. (Obviously, never while working, driving, or using any kind of machinery.) Your own bed is one natural choice, but anywhere you won't be interrupted for 20 minutes or so is OK.

STEP TWO: Relax. Lie down. Get comfortable. Close your eyes. Take three *deep* breaths. While you're exhaling the third breath, count silently to yourself, "Five, four, three, two, one." Imagine that each number brings you deeper into peaceful relaxation. Then say, silently, to yourself: "Relax now. Enjoy it. Get benefit from it."

STEP THREE: Relax more. After you've finished step two, just let yourself drift. If you don't feel completely relaxed yet—and you probably won't at first—try progressive relaxation: Feel the muscles in every part of your body, one part at a time, going limp and soft. Start with your head and work down to your feet. All the time, if stray thoughts pop into your head, just let them stay there as long as they want. Whatever you feel like daydreaming about is fine.

STEP FOUR: Think about your suggestion. When you're feeling relaxed, you can think about the reason you're doing the hypnosis—quitting smoking, cutting back on calories, or whatever you want to accomplish. The best way to do it is by thinking of all the benefits you'll achieve when you make the positive change you're working on.

STEP FIVE: Come back up. There's no time limit— stay in hypnosis as long as you want. About 20 minutes is typical. When you feel like coming back up, just say to yourself, "One, two, three, four, five." With each number, you gradually become more and more alert, awake. Then give yourself a minute or two to dust off the cobwebs before you go on with your business.

You don't have to have a specific change in mind in order to use this relaxation technique. Just getting yourself to relax a few times a day is a worthwhile end in itself. It's a great way to unwind.

Of course, hypnosis isn't a cure-all. Some problems, especially some psychological problems, should only be treated by a doctor or professional therapist. But hypnosis has its place. And that place is not on stage, making grown people bark like dogs.

When You Can't Sleep

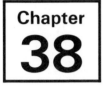

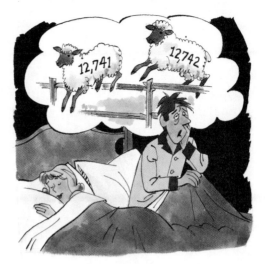

If counting sheep doesn't work for you,
there are some other cures for insomnia.

How did you sleep last night? Most people have occasional bouts of sleeplessness, and most of the time it's nothing to worry about. The amount of sleep we need varies, and our sleep patterns change as we get older. But for 25 million Americans, insomnia is an every-night curse. A lot of them turn to sleeping pills for relief, and some prescription medications *can* help lessen the effects of temporary insomnia. But when the pills are taken for more than a few days, they may end up making the sleeping problem worse than ever.

What causes insomnia? Not surprisingly, just about anything that can afflict a person during the day can create problems at night. When the problem is a passing one, such as a fight with a spouse or difficulty at work, the insomnia will clear up when the problem clears up. But when insomnia becomes chronic, it's time to examine the causes—the physical ones and the psychological ones.

Some of the more common physical causes include asthma, ulcers, migraine headaches, and angina (severe chest pain). In these cases the insomnia will clear up only when the diseases themselves are treated. Trying to overcome sleep problems related to serious physical ailments by taking sleeping pills may just create a drug dependence that makes it even harder to sleep than before—and it does nothing to treat the underlying cause.

One of the most serious sleep-related disorders is called sleep apnea. A person with this condition actually stops breathing for as long as a minute or more, and then awakens as the body tries to get air. The condition, though very rare, is life-threatening; in extreme cases the only solution is to surgically create a new breathing hole in the front of the neck in order to insure an unobstructed air passage.

Ironically, of all the psychological reasons for sleep difficulty, the toughest one to deal with may be the fear of not being able to sleep. Some people *think* they have insomnia when they are actually getting all the sleep they need. As we get older, we can get by on less sleep than we used to need. People in their 60's and 70's may do fine with only five or six hours a night.

If you're *not* getting the sleep you need, and the problem persists for more than a few nights, there are some remedies you can try:

• *Exercise.* There's nothing like good hard muscular exertion to put you in condition to sleep. Exercise helps ease the mental tension that may be keeping you awake. It's best not to exercise close to bedtime, though—that could be too stimulating.

• *Self-hypnosis.* You can learn how to hypnotize yourself by taking a course (check adult education programs). It's a lot like meditation, and it's a great way to relax the mind and body. (See Chapter 37.)

• *A warm bath.* Very soothing, and a good way to relax sore or stiff muscles.

• *A boring book.* Or a crossword puzzle, or some gentle music, or that old standby, the TV set.

• *Warm milk.* Once again, grandmother's advice turns out to be right. A glass of warm milk right before bed does indeed help you get to sleep. It turns out that one of the amino acids in milk has a sedative effect.

• *Avoid alcohol and caffeine.* Don't drink beverages that contain caffeine (coffee, tea, colas) after lunch if you're having a problem getting to sleep. As for alcohol, it may make falling asleep easier, but it shortens the sleep periods that the body needs most—the "rapid eye movement" (REM) sleep during which dreaming takes place.

• *Sex.* Some people become too stimulated to sleep after sex, but others find sex relaxing.

Sleeping pills are not the answer to insomnia. If you have trouble falling asleep, or you wake up during the night, or you find yourself awake before the alarm clock goes off, your body has a problem that requires careful treatment, the same as any other malady. Drugging yourself into unconsciousness is not a treatment. Even counting sheep is much better.

Laughter—Maybe It Really Is the Best Medicine

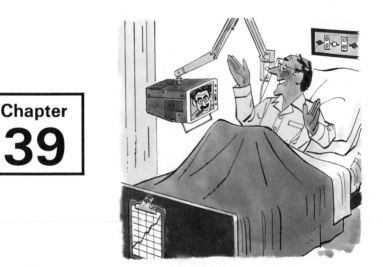

Chapter 39

Laughter has been called "the miracle drug with no bad side effects".

A merry heart doeth good like a medicine.
Proverbs 17:22

Comedy is one of man's most enduring ways of communicating. The ancient Greeks and Romans produced comedies. Shakespeare wrote comedies. Millions of TV watchers sit through hours of situation comedies. What is it about laughter that keeps everyone coming back for more?

These days, a lot of doctors and scientists are finding out that humor is good for more than selling theater tickets or building television ratings. Laughter, as the *Reader's Digest* has been reminding us for years, is the best medicine, and that medicine works in some surprising ways.

What happens when we laugh? A restrained giggle will make us feel good, but when we really cut loose in spasms of hilarity, the muscles of nearly every part of the body are exercised, even if only briefly. And believe it or not, that short burst of "exercise" is enough to do some good.

Research into laughter's beneficial effects is relatively new, but already some experts have become convinced that a good dose of the ho-ho-ho's can:

- improve digestion
- lower blood pressure
- stimulate the heart and circulatory system
- enhance creative thought
- soothe arthritis pain
- give the internal organs a workout
- speed recovery from disease.

When we laugh, we forget, if only for a moment, that we're uptight about something. The mere act of smiling seems to produce a chemical change in the body that soothes the troubled mind and calms the nerves. During a good, loud laugh, the pulse and blood pressure temporarily rise. But afterwards both pulse and blood pressure decrease—lower than before the laughter. Who knows—maybe one day doctors will tell their high-blood-pressure patients to read a few jokes and call them in the morning.

There's a scientific basis to all this. It has to do with substances called *endorphins*. Endorphins are, in effect, opiates made by the body. They have the same effect as the drugs people take to change their moods, block pain, or prevent depression. But endorphins are created naturally—there are no bad side effects to worry about. Vigorous exercise seems to stimulate the release of endorphins. So does meditation. And so does laughing.

Norman Cousins, the former magazine publisher and author of books about self-healing, has called laughter "internal jogging". He credits his sense of humor with helping him recover from a near-fatal degenerative spinal disease. Among the therapies he found helpful: watching Marx Brothers movies from his hospital bed.

Says Cousins: "I made the joyous discovery that ten minutes of genuine belly laughter had an anesthetic effect and would give me hours of pain-free sleep . . . . I was greatly elated to find that there is a physiologic basis for the ancient theory that laughter is good medicine."

Section VI - The "Little" Things

We know some cynics who have a standard come-back argument for not exercising, or for continuing to smoke, or for just ignoring all the advice they hear about health and fitness in general: "Why should I go to all that trouble to take care of my body, when I'll probably get killed in a car accident anyway?"

The answer to that one, of course, is that most people don't live their lives as if they have no control over them. And people who take care of themselves reap more than extra years for their efforts—they feel better for however many years they live.

Many people *will* die in car accidents, but it's not as if there's nothing you can do about that fate, either. Besides driving defensively and never drinking too much alcohol before driving, there are seatbelts. There's been a lot said about how much or how little good they do, and whether it's right for the government to require their use. We won't get into the requirement controversy. But there can be no doubt about seatbelts saving lives: they do.

In this section, we'll discuss some of the little things, like wearing seatbelts (Chapter 42), that can make a big difference. Next time you get a fever, you might want to follow the advice in Chapter 40. Or if you're heading for the beach to put on a golden tan, read Chapter 43 first. Chapter 45 is a reminder of the basics of dental care. Want to protect yourself against one of the most common ailments to which we desk jockeys are prone? Read about preventing back problems in Chapter 41. If you're one of the millions affected by a bad back, you know it's not such a "little thing" at all.

Fever: The Body's Germ Killer

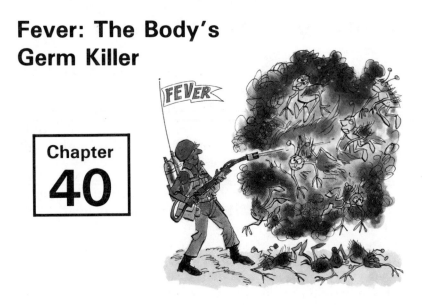

Chapter

40

Do you take pills when you have a fever? Your body has a better way.

Old-fashioned wisdom is often the best. Three hundred years ago, an English physician named Thomas Sydenham called fever "Nature's engine which she brings into the field to remove her enemy". And for hundreds of years before and after, the medical profession treated fevers as beneficial. But ever since the invention of aspirin about a hundred years ago, most doctors have advised their patients to bring down the fever.

At least until recently.

Now, there is a growing body of evidence that indicates Dr. Sydenham may have been right after all. Recent studies suggest that the best thing to do when you have a fever may be to allow it to run its course. Except for some people with heart conditions, and the very young and very old, a moderate fever is more likely to help you than hurt you.

The scientific explanation for this radical turnaround in medical thinking has to do with the way the body fights invading germs. Here's what happens:

1. When the body's immune system detects the presence of hostile bacteria or viruses, white blood cells are activated to surround and destroy the invaders.

2. These white cells release a hormone into the blood, called "endogenous pyrogen", which travels to the brain and acts on the body's internal "thermostat". Specifically, the EP raises the body's set point, so that the person now feels cold at a normally comfortable temperature.

3. Because the body now feels chilled, it fires up its furnace to raise the temperature—that is, it burns more fuel and causes the muscles to shiver, which produces heat. In the process, as many calories are burned up as if the person were involved in vigorous exercise—one reason people feel tired when they're sick. Other heat-producing behavior is stimulated as well—such as putting on warm clothes, drinking hot liquids, and climbing into bed with lots of covers.

4. The higher body temperature stimulates the production and release of two important elements of the immune system: T-cells, which help promote the growth of anti-bodies that attack the invaders; and interferon, a cellular substance that fights viruses (and is thought by some researchers to have anti-cancer potential).

5. The EP also drops the amount of iron in the blood. It

turns out that this effect is another weapon in the body's arsenal. When the body's temperature goes up, those invading germs need more iron to survive and reproduce. By dropping the iron level, the body helps kill the germs off.

This natural one-two punch, many doctors now believe, is a better way to fight viral or bacterial infection than by taking aspirin, aspirin substitutes, or antibiotics. There are, of course, some limits. Very high fever (say, above 101 degrees), or fever that lasts more than a day or two, is probably not good for you. And, as noted above, some people can't take the stress of fever as well as others.

But the benefits of higher-than-normal temperatures may explain something that joggers have been claiming for some time. Some joggers say that when they feel a bit sick, a good hard run cures them right away. And exercise is one of the surest ways of raising the body's internal temperature.

Next time the thermometer reads 100.8°, don't worry. It just means your body is fighting back.

Backache: Is It Inevitable?

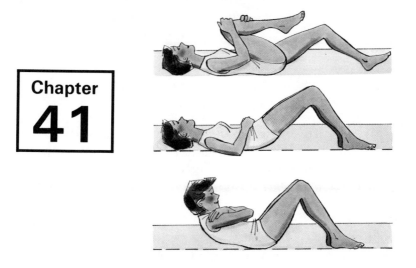

*Back problems affect 75 million Americans,
and cost billions.*

Back problems have something in common with heart disease and cancer: all are largely a result of the way we live today. In the case of heart disease and cancer, the major culprits are diet and smoking. The blame for back problems goes to several factors, including a sedentary lifestyle, poor posture, high-heeled shoes, improper lifting of heavy objects, a mattress that's too soft, poor sleeping position, and overweight. But even though there are many causes of backache, and even though this disease hits four out of five adults at some time or another, it's possible to significantly lower your risk.

Most back problems can be traced to weakness in the muscles of the back and abdomen rather than something going wrong with the bones or disks of the spine. So it stands to reason that strengthening those muscles is a good preventive step. The exercises pictured on page 151 are a good start; try to do them every day.

Top: Lie on your back with knees bent. Gently pull one knee toward your chin. Hold for count of ten, then release. Repeat with other leg. Work up to ten cycles.

Middle: Lie on your back with knees bent and feet on the floor. Pull in your stomach so that the small of your back presses on the floor. Tighten your buttocks and lift your hips off the ground. Hold for count of ten, then rest for count of five. Work up to 20 cycles.

Bottom: Lie on your back with knees bent and feet on the floor. Tuck your chin to your chest, and fold your arms across your chest. Raise your trunk off the floor about 30 degrees in a smooth motion, and return to starting position. Start with ten cycles, and work up to 50. For all exercises, it's important not to exceed your capabilities. If you experience pain, stop.

Other ways to protect your back:

1. *Lighten the load.* Three out of four people with back pain are overweight. The extra pounds that your back has to support put the spine under constant stress, and can lead to ruptured disks and muscle strain.

2. *Stand tall.* The way you stand can make a difference to your back. If you slouch, or allow your stomach to protrude, you exaggerate the curve of the lower spine, and that's not good. Instead, get in the habit of pulling in on your stomach (improves your appearance too!). When you have to stand for a long time, it helps to put one foot up on

the lower rung of a chair—it tilts your pelvis back and tends to flatten your back. It also helps if you shift positions from time to time.

3. *Sit in a good chair.* The best provide support to the lower back, are firm but comfortable, keep your knees slightly higher than your hips, and allow you to tilt and swivel.

4. *The fetal position.* Sleeping flat on your back or stomach can, believe it or not, put strain on the spine. The preferred position is on your side, with your knees bent— the "fetal position". What mattress? Firm is best.

5. *Lift with your legs.* To lift anything, squat down by bending your knees. Keep your back straight. Lift with your legs, not your back.

6. *No high heels.* Whatever fashion and tradition say, it's bad for your back to wear high heels—they add to the curve of the lower spine.

People with back problems should, of course, see a doctor to have them diagnosed and treated. Most back problems go away within a few months on their own—for a while. The human body is remarkable in its ability to adjust to all sorts of mistreatment. But the longer that mistreatment continues, the less likely the body's recovery becomes. The sooner you begin the preventive steps outlined here, the better. Back problems are common, costly, and painful. But they're not inevitable.

Are You That One In Ten?

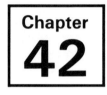

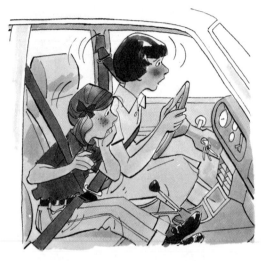

Most people <u>don't</u> wear seat belts. Maybe it's because they believe these myths.

Almost every car on the road today has seat belts. But only one person in ten uses them. How come? When you ask those other nine people why they don't use belts, it's almost like asking cigarette smokers why they smoke—everyone has a great reason.

Some people will never wear seat belts (just as some people will never quit smoking). But others might—if they just understood all the facts. What follows are some of the most frequently heard myths and misunderstandings about seat belts, and the truth.

Myth: Seat belts don't really do any good.

Fact: If you're in an accident, your chances of being

killed are twice as high if you're not wearing a seat belt.

Myth: Seat belts aren't necessary for local, low-speed driving.

Fact: Injuries, both minor and life-threatening, can and do happen at any speed. In one study, almost two-thirds of all injuries happened below 30 m.p.h. And three-fourths of all accidents are less than 25 miles from the driver's home.

Myth: If you wear a seat belt, you'll be trapped in a burning car.

Fact: The chances of fire, even in serious accidents, are less than one in five hundred. In those cases, seat belt wearers are usually in better condition to escape the fire than unbelted passengers.

Myth: Pregnant women shouldn't wear seat belts.

Fact: The greatest risk to an unborn child in the event of an accident is the death of the mother. And she is best protected by wearing a seat belt.

Myth: In an accident, you're better off being thrown clear of the car.

Fact: While there are rare instances of a person being saved because he or she was thrown from a car, your chances of severe injury or death are about 25 times higher if you're ejected. In a study of 177 crash fatalities, more than a quarter had been ejected. Most of them, it was found, would have lived if they'd been wearing belts.

Myth: Seat belts will fail in a serious crash.

Fact: Auto manufacturers are making seat belts more

reliable every year. The chances of seat belt failure are less than one in a hundred.

Myth: Seat belts are unsafe because they cause injuries.

Fact: In virtually every case where a seat belt caused an injury (a very rare occurrence), that injury was less serious than the ones it prevented. In order to minimize the risk, the lap belt should be worn like a bikini—at or below the protrusion of the hipbone. And both the lap and shoulder belt should always be used together.

Some people who don't use seat belts are acting more out of personal habit than out of misinformation. They say things like: "Seat belts are uncomfortable," or "I just never think of using them," or "I can't reach the radio with the belt on," or "I don't like to feel restrained."

We can't argue with these statements. If that's how they feel, no one can convince these people they're wrong. (As for never thinking of using belts, once it has become a habit, you don't have to think of it—you do it automatically.)

We just wonder if the people who make excuses for not wearing seat belts ever weigh those excuses against the one fact that matters more than all the rest—seat belts can cut your chances of death in an auto accident in half.

Is It Safe to Sun?

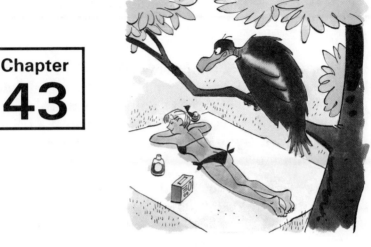

Chapter
43

More cancer is caused by exposure to the sun than by any other factor.

As many as half a million people get skin cancer every year, and most of them have the sun to blame. While most kinds of skin cancer are easily curable, thousands of people die. Is there any way to have your tan without paying the penalty?

Several decades ago, tanning wasn't the fashion it is now. Creamy white skin was a sign of wealth and sophistication. All that changed with America's growing love of the outdoors and exercise—we now equate tan skin with health and sexuality. But ask a dermatologist about this value system and you'll get a different story: Tan skin is damaged skin.

When the sun hits human skin, the skin burns. The

seriousness of that burn depends on several factors, including:

• *Skin type.* People who are light-skinned and have blond or red hair and blue or green eyes suffer the worst burning from the sun.

• *Angle of the sun.* The closer the sun is to directly overhead, the faster it burns you. And that angle is determined by the time of day (11 a.m. to 3 p.m. are the peak hours), time of year (summer sun burns faster than winter), and earth latitude (you'll burn faster in Florida than in Maine).

• *Exposure duration.* People with extremely sensitive skin can get a noticeable burn after only 10 or 15 minutes. For other people, it takes longer. But the longer you stay in the sun, the more you'll burn.

• *Protection.* There are several ways to protect yourself against sunburn. The most effective is to stay indoors, but who wants to spend the summer in front of the TV? Beyond that extreme, you can wear tightly-woven clothing, or use a parasol or umbrella, or stay in deep shade. If those measures still put too much of a crimp in your summer fun, and you're determined to get a tan, the best thing to use is a sunscreen.

Sunscreens are relatively new to the beach blanket arsenal. Ten years ago, the lotions and ointments that people were spreading on their skin provided about as much protection from the sun as a see-through bikini. Sunscreens, however, contain chemicals that block most of the sun's burning ultraviolet rays while allowing some of the tanning rays to get through. The screens won't *prevent* burning—they'll just allow you to stay in the sun longer before you burn.

But what about that tan—is there really a safe way to get one? The general answer is no—there is no 100 percent safe way to tan. Even if you manage to avoid getting skin cancer, the sun can hurt you in other ways. Each time you tan or burn, the fibers in your skin that keep it looking young and smooth are damaged. The result, after years of this kind of treatment, is what one doctor calls a complexion like a baseball glove.

We recognize, though, that no matter how dreadful the consequences sound, people still want that tan. So here are some guidelines that will at least minimize the hazards:

1. Start gradually—only 15 or 20 minutes for the first couple of times in the sun.

2. Avoid the peak hours.

3. Use a sunscreen—preferably one having a Skin Protection Factor of 10 to 15.

4. Don't count on a beach unbrella, or a cloudy sky, or light summer clothing, or a wide-brimmed hat to protect you from the sun. Most of the sun's ultraviolet rays get through.

5. Avoid sunbathing when taking certain drugs. Among the ones that can sensitize your skin are some antibiotics, birth control pills, diuretics, and tranquilizers.

Maybe what we really need is a change in society's idea of what's fashionable. Snow White had the right idea!

Eyes—Only Two to a Customer

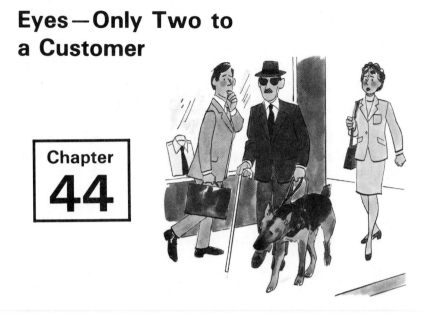

Chapter 44

Blindness is a tragedy. But there are some easy ways to prevent it.

If you're like most of the people reading this, you're probably saying to yourself, "Oh, no—another lecture about taking care of my eyes. I've heard it all before. Boring!" Well, there are *some* people who won't be saying that—anyone who has lost all or some eyesight, and anyone who *knows* someone with impaired vision. Blind and vision-impaired people are able to make remarkable adjustments to their handicap, but that doesn't make it any less a handicap.

The simple fact is, of all the five senses, eyesight is the one we can least afford to lose. The body does its part by protecting most of the eye in the skull, but eyes are still vulnerable in the front. In most cases, all it takes to protect that vulnerable part of the eyes is a pair of safety goggles.

Some of the hazards that eyes have to watch out for include:

Sports injuries. Eye doctors say there is an alarming increase in the number of people injured during participation in sports and recreational activities. Especially risky are tennis, baseball, hockey, racquetball, and squash. Does this mean you have to avoid these sports? Of course not. But safety experts urge that you wear protective goggles when you're participating in hazardous sports.

Fireworks. About a thousand people suffer eye injuries every year from fireworks. Others are luckier—they're "just" burned. Best advice (you know it already): Stay away from fireworks, and especially keep children away.

Power tools. For the most part, industry has done a great job of incorporating safety procedures into jobs that expose people to risk. It's probably the do-it-yourselfer working with a few electric tools or the home-owner mowing the lawn who's most likely to fail to take the necessary precautions. What a pity—it takes only a few seconds to put on safety goggles. Usually, that's all you have to do.

Chemicals and grooming aids. If you're spraying insecticide around the yard, you probably know you should protect your eyes from the poison. But you should really avoid getting *any* liquid, other than water or eye drops, in your eyes. When you use hair spray, close your eyes. When you use a paint sprayer, wear goggles.

Herpes. Herpes has become an epidemic in the U.S. It's

also a leading cause of blindness. If you have open herpes lesions (sores), don't touch them and then touch your eyes. If you accidentally *do* touch your eyes, see an ophthalmologist immediately. Proper medication can still save your eyes.

The sun. Overexposure to the sun is dangerous to your eyes, as well as to your skin. To protect your eyes from the sun's rays, wear sunglasses—preferably ones with polarized or mirrored lenses. To tell if a pair of sunglasses is dark enough to protect your eyes, put them on and look at yourself in a mirror. If you can't see your eyes, the glasses are dark enough.

Swimming pools. Most pools contain chlorine to kill bacteria, and some people are more sensitive to the chlorine than others. Too much chlorine can cause a mild burning of the eye's outer layer, a condition that usually clears up in a few days, but is quite painful in the meantime. Solution to the problem: Wear swim goggles.

When our eyes are working normally, we forget about them. But eyes, like any other part of the body, are subject to disease, and you should have yours checked by the ophthalmologist any time you suspect a problem. That's especially important for preschool kids, who may have problems you don't know about, and older people, who are more likely to come down with such eye problems as glaucoma and cataracts. In most cases, the earlier treatment is started, the better the chances of success.

If success means keeping the ability to watch the next gorgeous sunset, to witness the look on your child's face on Christmas morning, to follow a perfectly executed 70-yard punt return . . . a few simple preventive measures don't seem like such a burden, do they?

Look Ma—
No Cavities!

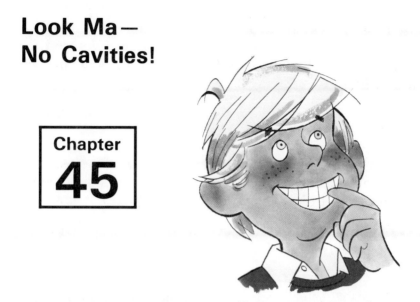

Chapter
45

Tooth decay is the nation's most common disease.
It's also one of the most preventable.

Dental caries—tooth decay—afflicts 98 percent of Americans. Every year it results in $8 billion in dental bills and the loss of 100 million hours of work. While tooth decay is rarely thought of in the way other, life-threatening diseases are, it has something very important in common with them. Prevention is a lot easier than cure. What *you* do to take care of your own teeth is what determines how healthy they are. And it's a lifetime occupation.

Everyone knows you should limit sweets. But what most people don't realize is that the kind of sweets and how and when they're eaten makes a big difference in how much damage they cause. The worst kind is anything sticky—like caramels, taffy, cookies, and pastry. Sweets eaten with meals do the least damage—partly because the rest of the meal helps dilute or brush away the sweets. And whatever and whenever you eat, if you can't brush right away, at least rinse your mouth with water.

When you do brush your teeth, there are a few hints to keep in mind.

• It's best to brush after every meal, but it's especially important to brush before you go to bed. Leaving food in the mouth overnight is an invitation to the worst damage.

• Avoid hard-bristled brushes—they can hurt the gums. Best are soft, flat-top brushes. Replace them every few months or so.

• Use a *fluoride* toothpaste that has been approved by the American Dental Association.

• At least once a day, use dental floss. It's something that many people forget, but it's almost as important as brushing.

While fluoride toothpaste will help prevent cavities, the addition of fluoride to the drinking water is even more effective. Fluoridation has been the subject of controversy in the past; some people have claimed various health dangers from fluoridated water. The charges have all been investigated and found to be groundless. Fluoride in drinking water is completely safe, and can reduce tooth decay by up to two-thirds.

Don't forget regular visits to the dentist for a cleaning and checkup. Twice a year is recommended. If you don't have a dentist, ask friends or neighbors to recommend one they know is good.

The most important thing to remember about taking care of your teeth is that it's *your* responsibility. It's not up to the dentist. He or she can give you advice, clean your teeth, and repair the damage when you have a cavity or need some other treatment. But nothing the dentist does is as important as the care you give your teeth every day.

Section VII - The Medical Profession

Some people treat their bodies the same as they treat their cars. Just as they drive until the family car breaks down—paying no heed to preventive maintenance—they pay no attention to their health until something happens to it. Then they run to the doctor, and expect him or her to "fix" them up.

Doctors are not gods. Another thing they're not is auto mechanics. There is no one in a better position to take care of your health than you. The doctor can help when something goes wrong, but you're the only one who can keep something from going wrong. It's your responsibility to keep the "machine" working the way the manufacturer intended.

In the last section of this book, we'll give you some guidelines for establishing a relationship with your doctor. The operative word here is "partnership". Doctors are specialists in curing and treating disease. But they can't keep you healthy without your cooperation. Of course, if you've been paying attention to the other chapters, you already know how to do that.

Choosing and Using a Doctor: A Quiz

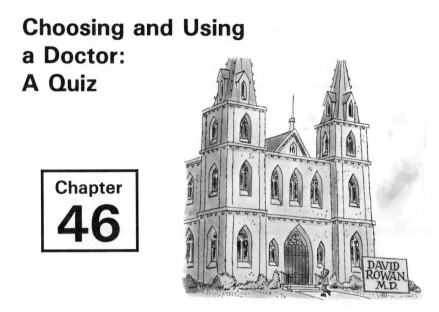

Most people are either in total awe, or total fear of doctors.

How much do you know about picking a good doctor, and knowing how to deal with him or her? Here's a quiz to help you find out.

1. The best time to find a doctor is:

    a. when you're sick.
    b. when you need a fourth for golf.
    c. when you're feeling fine.

2. The best kind of doctor to choose for your personal physician is:

    a. a gynecologist, if you're a woman.
    b. an orthopedist, if you have problems with your joints.

c. an eye/ear/nose/throat doctor, if you frequently have head colds.
   d. a general practitioner or internist.

3. Your doctor should ideally be:

   a. very old and very wise.
   b. very young and energetic.
   c. somewhere in between.

4. The qualifications you should look for in a doctor include:

   a. graduation from a good medical school.
   b. certification by specialty boards.
   c. association with a nearby, quality hospital.
   d. good reputation among the community.

5. When the doctor uses a term you don't understand, you should:

   a. write it down, and look it up in the dictionary when you get home.
   b. nod politely as if you understood.
   c. ask what it means.

6. When you disagree with something your doctor has suggested, you should:

   a. follow the doctor's advice—that's what you're paying for.
   b. get a second opinion.
   c. do what *you* think is right.
   d. tell the doctor why you disagree.

7. If you're embarrassed to discuss sensitive problems with the doctor, you should:

a. not discuss them.
b. discuss them in vague, general terms.
c. do it anyway.

8. The pills your doctor has prescribed don't seem to help. You should:

a. try a lower dose.
b. stop taking them for a few days.
c. tell the doctor.

Answers

For all but #4, the best answer is the last choice. For #4, all answers are right.

We hope this not-very-difficult quiz has started you thinking about your relationship with the medical profession. If you don't have a personal physician, there's no better time to begin finding one than when you're feeling fine. You should take the time to find someone you'll feel comfortable with—and confident in.

That confidence, though, shouldn't keep you from speaking up whenever you have a question. Doctors don't want to be worshipped—they want patients who take an active part in their own health. Sometimes that means doing exactly what the doctor orders. But sometimes it means first making sure the order is the right one.

The Annual Physical: Too Much of a Good Thing?

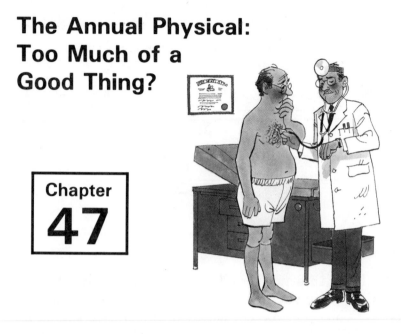

Chapter
47

Most people can get by without a complete checkup every year.

When you think about it, it really doesn't make sense. What's so special about a one-year period? Why is a complete physical exam necessary once every year—why not once every 512 days? Or every two months?

Aside from making it easier for people to remember that it's time to go see the doctor, there *is* no compelling medical need for an annual physical. At least not *complete* physicals, and not for everyone. Regular checkups do serve a purpose, of course—they get people to think about their health. And some diseases, notably cancer and heart disease, are easier to treat and cure if caught at their early stages. But more and more doctors have become convinced that healthy adults can afford to be selective about the amount of medical probing they put themselves through.

For example . . .

• *Blood-pressure test.* A simple, inexpensive, painless procedure that takes only a minute or two and can reveal an otherwise hidden case of hypertension. If you don't want to go to the doctor for this test, you can buy a sphygmomanometer of your own and check your own BP. For people under 40, though, unless your pressure exceeds about 130/90, a test about once every five years is sufficient. After 40, or if your pressure (or a close relative's pressure) is high, have the test every one to three years.

• *Cancer detection.* Tests for *colon and rectal cancer* probably are not necessary before age 50, but should be annual after that. The *chest X-ray* has fallen into disfavor as a method of detecting lung cancer and other respiratory diseases. Most doctors feel that the radiation hazard it imposes outweighs any possible benefits. Women have always been told to have an annual *Pap test,* and the test is without question an effective way of detecting cervical cancer. But once every three years is enough, says the American Cancer Society. *Mammograms* should be taken once before age 40 and every one to two years thereafter, and should be supplemented by monthly breast self-examination.

• *Hearing and vision tests.* For people who notice no obvious problems, regular testing probably is unnecessary before 40; once every five years thereafter is sufficient. One exception: A *tonometry test* for glaucoma should be performed every two or three years past age 40.

• *Blood count and urinalysis.* Once every three to five years, except for people with a family history of diabetes.

Doctors have tests for just about every part of the body, and most of the time those tests won't do you any harm— other than the expense. But study after study has failed to prove that normal, healthy adults improve their odds of preventing disease by having these tests every year.

For people who are at higher-than-average risk, however, the tests make more sense. Those people include anyone with a family history of cancer, heart disease, diabetes, or hypertension; people who themselves have one of these diseases; and people whose lifestyles increase their chances of health problems—lifestyles such as smoking, excessive alcohol, being overweight, getting no aerobic exercise, and regular contact with hazardous substances on the job.

Does all this spell the end of the complete annual physical? Probably not. Many people will conclude that it's too much trouble to figure out which tests to have performed, or they'll "play it safe", and continue to tell the doctor they want "the works".

Others will recognize that their health is their own responsibility, not the doctor's. That concept would have been considered radical a while back. But it's catching on. It's one reason Americans are healthier today than they've ever been before. And it's the subject of our final chapter.

Your Health,
Your Responsibility

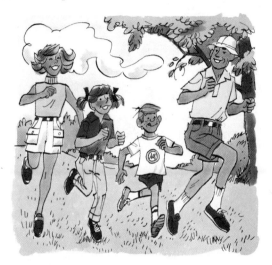

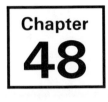

*Doctors can <u>restore</u> good health, but only you
can <u>maintain</u> it.*

It used to be that the only time people thought about
their health was when they lost it. If you got sick, you
went to the doctor. The doctor prescribed a pill, you took
the pill, you got well. And then you put the subject of
health out of your head.

That's the way it still works for a lot of people, but
things are changing for millions of others. The health
and fitness movement has put some pretty radical ideas
into the national consciousness, and one of them is the
notion that we are responsible for our own health.

It's something like the concepts of war and peace.
Peace is not just the absence of war, it's a way of living

that demands constant effort. Likewise, health is not just how you are between illnesses—health is what you have when you do the right things for yourself. Illness is what you have when you *don't*.

What are those right things? (Haven't you been paying attention to the rest of the book?) Here's a brief review:

• At the top of the list is *avoiding cigarette smoke*. No single measure has a greater impact on health and long life than not smoking.

• *Use common sense in the consumption of alcohol and food*. This means that your normal pattern is to have no more than one or two drinks a day, to eat a balanced diet that contains plenty of fiber, vitamins, and minerals, and to eat only enough calories to maintain your proper weight. An occasional excess is no big deal, as long as it's really occasional.

• *Use your muscles*. Bodies fall apart faster if they're not used. Watching TV and driving a car are two examples of not using your body. The more you move, the better. It all has to do with strengthening the most important muscle, the heart.

• *Drive with belts*. All the excuses for not wearing seatbelts—they're too uncomfortable, not really effective, not necessary for short trips, or just too much trouble to remember—don't change the simple fact that seatbelts could save 25,000 American lives a year—if Americans wore them.

• *Know how to unwind*. Stressful job or home life? It doesn't have to give you an ulcer or high blood pressure. Exercise is a great way to dissipate tension. The best exercises are the ones that get you breathing hard and work up a sweat.

• *When you need to, see a doctor.* Taking responsibility for your own health doesn't mean treating doctors as the enemy. It means treating them as your partners. Sometimes, for whatever reason, you need their help. It may be for preventive measures—immunizations, advice on a weight-reducing diet or exercise program, or help in quitting smoking. Or it may be to diagnose a problem you've found, such as a lump or a persistent cough. And when you get sick, the doctor may be the *only* one who can help.

But too many people are counting on the doctor to undo the damage they cause by lifelong neglect. Why worry about smoking or cholesterol, they figure. If I get heart disease, I'll just have a bypass operation, or a transplant, or take pills. If I get cancer, well, they're curing more and more these days, and anyway, we all have to go sometime.

It's true that modern medicine has come up with some marvelous weapons for combatting serious diseases. But they don't work all the time, they cost a lot of money, and no cure is ever as good as prevention.

Good health doesn't mean avoiding all the things that are fun. It means finding out how you can have fun and treat your body right at the same time. Anyone who has "converted" to healthful living will tell you: It's not just a matter of adding years to your life. You'll be adding life to your years.